AIDS

Anne Aaron
Iben Browning

Sapiens Press
a division of Joy Inc.

Albuquerque, NM

COPYRIGHT © 1988 by SAPIENS PRESS

ALL RIGHTS RESERVED. NO PART OF THIS BOOK MAY BE REPRODUCED OR TRANSMITTED IN ANY FORM OR BY ANY MEANS, ELECTRONIC OR MECHANICAL, INCLUDING PHOTOCOPYING, RECORDING, OR ANY INFORMATION STORAGE AND/OR RETRIEVAL SYSTEM, WITHOUT WRITTEN PERMISSION FROM SAPIENS PRESS.

SAPIENS PRESS
a division of Joy Inc.
2430 Juan Tabo NE
Suite 256
Albuquerque, NM 87112

Library of Congress Cataloging in Publication Data

ISBN 0-945904-08-8

PRINTED IN THE UNITED STATES OF AMERICA
1 2 3 4 5 6 7 8 9

To Our Grandchildren

Crystal

Jimmy
Jeannie

You undoubtedly will be touched
by the AIDS pandemic, but...

May You Survive.

CONTENTS
FOREWORD viii
PREFACE x
ACKNOWLEDGEMENT. xii

PART I: ECONOMIC SURVIVAL AND AIDS
  WORK 3
  ALL GOODS AND SERVICES REQUIRE WORK 3
  ALL GOODS AND SERVICES ARE LIMITED 4
    Hidden Economic Impacts of AIDS 4
  WORK IS LIMITED 8
    Nutrition and AIDS 10
  ALL BUDGETS ARE LIMITED: YOURS,
  BUSINESSES' AND GOVERNMENT'S 11
  AIDS Costs 12
  AIDS VIRUS - THE ENEMY 15
  AFRICAN AIDS: Mirror for our Future AIDS 17
  IMPACT OF AIDS ON THE FAMILY ECONOMY .. 19
    Lack of Supportive Families 20
  OUR BASIC ECONOMIC ASSUMPTIONS 21
    All Economies Are Limited 21
    Working People=Work=People's Supply 21
    Work = Supply 23
    No Work = No Supply, sooner or later 24
  ALL ECONOMIES ARE LIMITED 25
    Moving Families 26
    Working Women 26
    Breakup of Nuclear Families 27
    Burying the Dead 27
    High Cost of Dying of AIDS 28
    No Home for Many 28
  SUBTLE BUT VERY REAL IMPACT OF AIDS 29
    Education and Art 29
    Less of Everything 30
    Measure of Humanity 30

CONTENTS

OUR PRESENT ECONOMIC SITUATION
(Some Say It Is Better, We Do Not Agree) 32
Family Purchasing Power 33
National Economy and Family Budgets 34
INCREASING MEDICAL DEMANDS/DECREASING RESOURCES 35
AIDS IMPACT WILL NOT BE EQUAL 40
Major Metropolitan Areas Will Be Hit First 40
Specific Minorities Will Increase Their
AIDS Proportions 48
The Impact Will Be Astounding 53
A SPECIAL GROUP: RETIREES 53
Social Security 54
Present and Future Retirees 54
Lost Liquidity 56
Future Social Security Problems 58
Our Increasingly Older Population 58
Why People Are Not Saving Enough for
Retirement.....60
Attitudes on Pensions and Retirement 62
Medicare 67
IMPACT OF AIDS ON BUSINESS AND WORKERS 70
Public Fear of AIDS 72
Insurance Costs 76
Lost Productivity 83
Business and Occupations Affected by AIDS 85
Company AIDS Policies 88
Conclusion 93

PART II: THE SCIENCE OF AIDS
MAN 99
THE AFFLICTION 101
WHAT IS AIDS? 102
PHASE I 103

CONTENTS

AIDS Antibodies Test 104
Unknown Transmission Modes 107
AIDS and the Young 110
PHASE II 111
PHASE III 115
    The Complexity of the AIDS Virus 115
    Humility Not Hubris 116
PHASE IV 118
CONCLUSIONS 119
THE HISTORY OF AID 120
DISCUSSION 128
    Coping With AIDS 130
    A Short History of Plagues 131
    A Philosopher's Thoughts 133
    Diagnostics 137
    Other Efforts to Cope 139
    AIDS Cases 140
    More Evidence 141
CONCLUSIONS 142
APPENDICES
    (A) CORPORATE SECURITY & INVESTIGATIONS,
        INC. Designing a Corporate AIDS Policy 14
    (B) CHEVRON, January 1986 15
    (C) THE BANK OF AMERICA, October 1985 15
REFERENCES - PART I 15
REFERENCES - PART II 16

LIST OF TABLES - PART I
TABLE I   AIDS DEATHS (Death Graphs) 1
TABLE II SOURCES OF RETIREMENT INCOME
        1962 AND 1984 5
TABLE III SOURCES OF 1984 AGGREGATE INCOME
        FOR THOSE AGED 65 AND OVER 56
TABLE IV WHY PEOPLE ARE PUTTING NO MONEY
        OR NOT ENOUGH MONEY ASIDE FOR
        RETIREMENT 61

CONTENTS

TABLE V ADEQUACY OF STANDARD OF LIVING AMONG RETIREES 62
TABLE VI AMOUNT OF PLANNING FOR RETIREMENT 62
TABLE VII RETIREMENT PLANNING AND INCOME ADEQUACY 64
TABLE VIII AMOUNT OF PLANNING FOR RETIREMENT 64
TABLE IX ANY THOUGHT GIVEN TO AMOUNT OF MONEY REQUIRED AFTER RETIREMENT. 65
TABLE X LOST PRODUCTIVITY 84
TABLE XI AMERICAN WAR DEAD 91
TABLE XII AIDS INFECTIONS IN THE UNITED STATES AND UNITED KINGDOM 95

LIST OF TABLES - PART II

TABLE A WEIGHT & LIFE SPANS OF VARIOUS ANIMALS AND MAN 99
TABLE I   FATALITIES 102
TABLE II   NAMES OF AIDS 104
TABLE III AIDS TRANSMISSION MODES 106
TABLE IV AIDS RELATED DISEASES 108
TABLE V   KAPOSI'S SARCOMA 109
TABLE VI   DEATH IN STATES 113
TABLE VII POPULATION GROUPINGS 114
TABLE VIII NEW YORK AIDS DEATHS 125
TABLE IX   AIDS TEST ON 306,061 MIL. RECRUITS .. 126
TABLE X WHITES, BLACKS, HISPANICS 128
TABLE XI TRANSMISSION PROBABILITY 128

LIST OF FIGURES - PART II

FIGURE 1 WEIGHTS & LIFE EXPECTANCY IN YRS .. 100
FIGURE 2 DEAD FROM AIDS 112

FOREWORD

This timely book brings two sobering messages to the American people. The first is concerned with the possibility that the AIDS epidemic may very well become the "Black Plague" of the 21st century. The second is that the future economic costs of AIDS may be devastating to our society. The AIDS epidemic, in short, carries the potential for both health and economic disaster.

The authors destroy the commonly held myth that only homosexuals, prostitutes, and needle-using drug addicts are the main victims. They suggest that the AIDS epidemic is a time bomb ready to explode, since minorities living in inner-city ghettos and sexually-active teenagers are high risk candidates to become afflicted with the disease. The socio-economic implications of this finding are explosive, to say the least, since there is a potential for the AIDS epidemic to spread at a geometric rate at a time when no known medical cure exists.

Given these stark realities, the authors conclude that education to promote intelligent preventative measures is the cutting edge of the battle against AIDS. Time is of the essence.

The fundamental problem, however, lies in the attitudes of a society riddled with social stigmas, taboos, ignorance, inertia, scientific limits, lack of awareness and caring, and the fiscal mythologies of the Reagan legacy—all of which work against finding timely solutions to the problem and adequate care for the afflicted.

Having researched the stark realities of the health and economic implications of the AIDS epidemic, the authors conclude that this is a story with neither a beginning nor an ending. They conclude, further, that there lies a great distance between the *reality* of the problem and the *answers* which will prevent a human "meltdown" during the next several decades.

Insofar as public education is the main weapon for the prevention of AIDS in the near term, it is sensible to conclude that an ounce of prevention today is worth a pound of cure in a distant future.

FOREWORD

The message of the book is clear, namely, that the critical moment has arrived when we all must become more deeply involved in a dialogue and the public policy programs currently addressing the AIDS epidemic.

Gerhard N. Rostvold, Ph.D.

PREFACE

AIDS was written for everyone who reads. Our particular emphases are on AIDS transmission and the impact AIDS will have on all of our economic lives. AIDS will hit employees and employers alike. AIDS will affect consumers and suppliers in ways never before seen. Laws will be changed. Government expenditures will shift due to the massive economic burdens created by AIDS.

And you never have to contract AIDS to have you life severely impacted by AIDS. Not only are we faced with supporting those dying from AIDS, but we are also going to face a significant decline in the real numbers of our most productive workers. Those dying of AIDS will be somewhere between 20-50 years old. The younger and older members of our population will be forced to support our nonworking youngest and oldest members.

To prevent AIDS from devastating all of us, some apparent issues must be addressed now. For instance, care fo an AIDS patient can cost up to $175,000, but in San Francisco costs have been brought down to about $30,000 per year. In most future cases, society will have to share in the cost burden. Whether the state through welfare assumes the cost or someone's medical insurance covers treatment, you and I ultimately share the cost. In fact, because so many insurance companies also serve as investment companies for retirement plans, AIDS costs may affect you in ways that you have never considered.

Your family members, friends, fellow workers, employees, and even enemies need to know and protect themselves, too, as you will soon learn. But it may surprise you to learn that it is not just contact with the AIDS virus from which you need to protect yourself and others. The AIDS virus will so profoundly affect everyone's social and economic lives that we had better start some protective measures in those areas now.

PREFACE

We further need to say something about the "style" of this book. Each author wrote separate Parts. Aaron wrote "Part I: Economic Survival and AIDS." Browning wrote "Part II: The Science of AIDS." Each author supports what the other wrote.

However, when you read <u>AIDS</u>, you will discover that our syntax and styles of writing are different. You may further notice that one of us tends to be more socially liberal and the other more socially conservative. (Both of us are fiscally conservative.) We have made no attempt to force our opinions to agree.

Our separate analyses of available AIDS data led us to agree on the contents of this book. We believe that liberals and conservatives alike will also agree, though none of us will be pleased by the consequences of AIDS.

There is no doubt that healthy-mindedness is inadequate as a philosophical doctrine, because the evil facts which it positively refuses to account for are a genuine portion of reality; and they may after all be the best key to life's significance, and possibly the only openers of our eyes to the deepest levels of truth. (William James, 1958.)*

We have chosen to present "the evil facts." We ask our readers to exercise their own judgements.

Anne Aaron
Iben Browning

---

*William James, <u>The Varieties of Religious Experience.</u> (New York: Mentor, 1948), pp. 137-138.

ACKNOWLEDGMENTS

We want to thank the following people:

Joseph Cotruzzola, The Business Editor of Sapiens Press, who led us to new information and insights;

Florence Browning, who makes life worth living for many;

Michael Sutin, whose acumen led us to risk but cut material;

Esther Sutin, whose art has constant sensitivity and depth; and

Gerhard Rostvold, Ph.D., who comprehends human as well as abstract economics.

LIMRA

Life Insurance Marketing and Research Association, Inc.
Dorothy F. Murray, Scientist/Project Director
The Retirement Markets: Overview and Outlook
8 Farm Springs
Farmington, CT 06032

Corporate Security and Investigations, Inc.
Evelyn Garriss, Research Director for
Designing a Corporate AIDS Policy
700 Silver, SW
Albuquerque, NM 87102
Other offices in Millis, MA and New York, NY
1-(800)-443-3119

PART I: ECONOMIC SURVIVAL AND AIDS

WORK

Even if you are economically sophisticated, we ask you to read this initial section of our economic discussion. We thoroughly examined our economic assumptions regarding the effects AIDS will have on our economy. Then we simplified those assumptions to the very basics.

We begin Part II with what we regard as the most fundamental aspects of any and all economies. Although at first our discussion may not seem directly related to AIDS, we will refer to our underlying economic assumptions throughout Part II: Economic Survival and AIDS.

ALL GOODS AND SERVICES REQUIRE WORK

Most families in Western countries have not yet been perceptibly touched by the economic effects of AIDS. Some of us know a friend who had a family member or friend who had AIDS and died of AIDS. Some of us know someone with ARC. (The authors believe that the difference between AIDS and ARC is merely definitional. If a person has ARC, his disease will progress to the point of being defined as AIDS.) Anyone who reads or watches TV has read about, heard about, and/or seen people with AIDS.

But at this point, it all seems so remote, so impersonal. Nonetheless, AIDS costs are already affecting everyone's life and life style.

All goods and services are limited - because supply is limited - because work is limited. Every dollar directly or indirectly spent on AIDS affects supply. Every work hour used to support AIDS costs simply means that the work hour cannot be spent producing some other type of supply.

Money (particularly money without a concrete standard such as the old gold standard) is nothing more than a convenient way to transfer or exchange work. When we buy a suit, that may not be very obvious. After all, a suit hanging silently on a rack does not look too much like work. The money or credit card we use to purchase the suit does not look too much like work either. But our work, or someone's work, earned the money to buy the suit. Work produced the suit, distributed the suit, and sold the suit to the retailer who will now work and sell the suit to us.

A suit is a good example of forgotten work. If someone(s) did not gather the wool or cotton or polymerize complex esters, those would remain in nature. People then have to process those materials, make yarn, weave the yarn, dye the yarn somewhere along the way, invent a pattern, cut the yarn-now-fabric, sew the fabric—using buttons and zippers that also require long work processes to develop—press the suit, sell the suit to a wholesaler who then sells it to a retailer who then sells the suit to you. And even in this description, we have failed to mention a lot about the work required to make and get a suit to a consumer.

Because we buy finished products and services, the work involved is often forgotten. It can be a 2 x 4, car part, or suit; each is a finished product. Some finished products such as a 2 x 4 may end up in another finished product, but that does not change the fact that work is requisite to produce any finished product. The information that we buy and the food service we receive in a restaurant are also finished work products.

We do not want to belabor the point. We hold that all goods and services require work. Money is only a convenient transfer mode for exchanging work. But we need to be mindful of that, for every dollar spent on AIDS anything will reduce the available dollars elsewhere.

ALL GOODS AND SERVICES ARE LIMITED
ALL GOODS AND SERVICES REQUIRE WORK

Hidden Economic Impacts of AIDS

While a suit for sale in a store can remind us of forgotten work, all sorts of impacts on other work products may be hidden until we dig out information. AIDS is and will continue to have a tremendous influence on many types of work products.

For instance, you are probably seeing the last fashion wave promoting short skirts. As sexual mores change, those changes are reflected in fashion trends. Sexual standards are becoming more constrained, and that will show up in persons' clothing choices.

When thigh-high skirts drop to mid-calf, about 1/3 more fabric, 1/10 more thread, and 1/10 more labor are required. Due to the effect of AIDS on sexual standards, such fashion changes will occur. Business, in turn, will be affected. Increased material and labor costs will impact the economy. Those changes will affect every economic sector - family, business, and national productivity.

We have no way of knowing how much something like AIDS-caused fashion changes will influence other sectors of our economy. The effects will be both direct and indirect, however. For example, as people cover their skin more with clothing, will they perspire more? Will discretion lead to perspiration? If so, deodorant sales will increase. AIDS is impacting and will continue to impact our economy in many generally unrecognized ways. You can be sure, though, that the costs are, or will be, passed to all of us.

All investors, large or small, need to examine thoroughly any and all investment opportunities. Without examining all investment data with traditional analyses and then including the entirely new economic information about the impact of AIDS, investors will lose money, the fruits of their work.

When we examine possible business trends, we need to watch out for what we call economic seesaw investments. A seemingly obvious good investment may not turn out to be such a good investment at all when we look at further information and extrapolate from that information.

A drug company developing an inexpensive blood test that directly tests for the AIDS virus rather than the AIDS antibodies may be a good investment. Certainly, the drug company that develops the first cheap AIDS viral test will have a market edge. Stock values in such a company can soar.

If we only partially research that drug company, however, we can make some really poor investment decisions. The drug company that develops the first cheap, effective AIDS viral test will have an edge. Is the management and distribution system in place to keep up with demand and get the AIDS viral tests to using markets?

Let us assume that the drug company has (1) the first inexpensive, effective AIDS viral test, and (2) the management and distribution system in place. The possibly critical question has not been asked: (3) Is the drug company pouring all or much of its profits into its research and development department, trying to develop effective AIDS treatment and cure drugs?

If that is the case, the drug company is not a good stock investment. The drug company will only be trapped on the economic seesaw - great profits from AIDS viral tests/great losses from unsuccessful AIDS treatment and cure drug developments. The research and development costs will simply crash down so hard that those R & D costs will flip the profits off the high side of the company's economic seesaw.

Presently, "The Food and Drug Administration has given priority to more than 40 anti-AIDS drugs involved in more than 100 human studies in the USA. Corporate USA now sponsors most of the publicly known studies." "Potential reward: More than $1 billion in sales." (Rebello, 1988)[1]

The authors are convinced that there will be little profits connected to those research and development costs and AIDS drug sales. AIDS is and will continue to be like cancer: We have poured billions into cancer research for decades. No cure for cancer exists; no vaccine has been developed that is effective against cancer. We are and will continue to pour billions into AIDS research in the coming decades. No cure for AIDS will be found; no vaccines will be developed that are effective against AIDS.

It does not matter that such eminent research scientists as Dr. Jonas Salk, who developed our polio vaccine, are attempting to develop an AIDS vaccine. Compared to the AIDS virus, the polio virus is a simple and predictable virus. As we have already discussed, AIDS is much more similar to cancer viruses. Furthermore, AIDS is mutating faster than anything any and all research scientists have ever seen.

> The HIV virus is constructed to evade the immune response. So it is not enough just to boost the immune system. This doesn't bode well for vaccine research. (Tertmiller, quoted by Krieger, 1987)[2]

Drug companies will not have the only dead end investment side. Other companies directly dealing with AIDS will experience the brick walls and over-weighted cost sides of their own economic seesaws. Still other companies that have no direct business with AIDS will have their own economic balance upset by the impact of AIDS.

Investors who do not burn the night oil and do their investment homework will be toppled off as AIDS costs slam one side of the seesaw down. Those who recognize the huge impact that AIDS will have on everything from single stocks to the overall economy will survive best economically - their limited work will continue to have value rather than being thrown away to no productive end.

Promiscuity is the swamp of AIDS. When we examine the proportion of needle-using drug addicts, hemophiliacs, and persons receiving AIDS infected blood transfusions, they are about equivalent to the flower pots and ditches that were drained in the Panama Canal in early attempts to control malaria. Just draining the flower pots and ditches would have had little effect on the mosquitoes spreading malaria. The major breeding ground of mosquitoes - swamps - had to be drained. Eliminating problems of blood passed through needles would have about the same effect on the spread of AIDS as draining flower pots and ditches has had on the spread of malaria. The promiscuous swamp of AIDS must be drained.

Bednets and screens did and continue to help prevent the spread of malaria because the mosquitoes are prevented from infecting people. Condoms do not prevent the sexual spread of AIDS. They are about as effective against AIDS as putting up bednets and screens with foot-large holes would be against mosquito-carried malaria.

We offer our analogy to discuss business investments. Condom sales will continue because they can be effective against other things. However, present condom sales will never be as high as they would have been if they had also been effective against the sexual spread of AIDS.

If we only examine the business market to this level, we will miss an area of business that will substantially increase as AIDS spreads. Not only condoms but also "rubber" gloves are made from latex. Latex is dissolved by oil products. But if janitorial people wear latex gloves without lotion or cream, latex gloves will offer janitors protection as they are cleaning restrooms, as the British know.

Medical and janitorial use of latex gloves will substantially increase sales of latex and latex gloves. Medical personnel wear disposable latex gloves, and janitors in England wear heavy latex gloves. Cleaning persons in the U.S. will wear heavy latex gloves that require a lot of latex for each set of gloves.

We may see another type of economic seesaw effect with raw latex: Latex sales will decline as latex condom sales decline/latex sales will increase as latex glove sales increase. Soon we should be able to determine the overall trend for latex sales. We will see similar trends in other business areas. Whatever the business, however, we need to include AIDS impacts in any of our business analyses.

Any business needs to ask itself how AIDS can directly or indirectly affect that business. Any investor also needs to ask himself/herself the same question. Those who settle for shallow answers will get bounced off the economic seesaw. Work will be wasted.

Work for manufacture and sales of condoms to prevent AIDS is wasted because condoms do not afford AIDS protection part of the time. In fact, we not only waste our national work supply, but also increase the death rate among our sexually active, most work productive age group. This is a lose-lose deal. We lose the work-earned savings; we lose part of our working population.

It is not just tomorrow's investments that are being poured down the drain. Families', businesses', and government's investments are being thrown away now because adequate planning, research, and extrapolation have not been done. The work (productivity) that provided the investment funds is being wasted. Up in smoke like a burnt house, once that productive work is gone, it is gone forever.

And it is not just the research and development projects and seesaw investments that are wasting a lot of our earned, or to be earned, productive work. When we examine the costs for caring for AIDS victims, the cost variations are astounding.

San Francisco has done an amazing job of lowering the economic care costs for AIDS victims while continuing to treat those people humanely. By using San Francisco's treatment programs as models, other cities would discover that they do not have to "re-invent the wheel." San Francisco has already done much of the research for them. Through far less costly extrapolation from those AIDS treatment programs, cities could save a lot of the taxpayers' tax dollars.

When AIDS victims can no longer work, his/her productive work input to our overall economy is gone. When research and development efforts produce nothing effectual, not only the R & D work is gone, but also the savings that came from work that supported the R & D investment is gone. The same is true of seesaw investments. When tax dollars are wasted, they are gone. All those tiny to huge work suppliers are permanently gone: AIDS victims - dead; work-savings for R & D and seesaw investments - gone, having produced little or nothing; work dollars for tax dollars spent on far-too-high costs.

It does not matter how far back we have to go in the chain of a supply of anything. We will always find that everything economic requires work. Anytime work is wasted or someone dies, a supply source is permanently gone from our economy. That loss affects anyone living in our economic system. Nationally, the AIDS related work losses are so small that very few of us have even noticed the work-loss impacts. We all will.

WORK IS LIMITED
WHEN WORK IS GONE,
WORK IS PERMANENTLY GONE

In larger cities in which AIDS is most prevalent, citizens are already beginning to experience increasing tax burdens for AIDS education and care. In certain businesses such as the fashion industry, AIDS deaths are already affecting work production. In offices and plants where AIDS victims are working, production is being affected by the uninformed panic of fellow workers. Directly and indirectly, work efficiency, production, and savings are being destroyed, never to be regained.

Panic has already caused human suffering and property damage. Social reactions to AIDS are causing economic losses. "Likewise, educators and business managers tell of disruptions, grievances and pressures to institute ill-founded screening programs and to isolate infected individuals so that the 'perceived risk' to others is eliminated." (Walters, 1987)[3]

Exactly what on-the-job disruptions are presently costing our economy, no one knows. However, everyone researching AIDS-caused job disruptions and worker time spent on the job worrying about AIDS agrees that AIDS has become a real and costly employment issue.

An early 1988 study by the Center for Work Performance at the Georgia Institute of Technology points to the problems of panic.

> "If a company can expect 35 to 40 per cent of its work force to be afraid of using the cafeteria or to refuse to share equipment, that has serious implications," Herold said. [David Herold is the director of the Center.]
>
> It [the Georgia Tech survey] found that 66 per cent of those who responded said they would be 'concerned' about using the same restroom on the job as the person who had acquired immune deficiency syndrome.
>
> Forty per cent said they would think twice about eating in the same cafeteria as an AIDS patient, while 37 per cent said they would not share tools or equipment with such a person. (Associated Press, 1988)[4]

Some time ago the author Jean-Paul Sartre said, "Hell is other people." With AIDS, that is proving to be true.

While writing this book, we interviewed over a hundred people - everyone from AIDS researchers and scientists to everyday workers. It did not matter to whom we spoke; everyone interviewed was deeply concerned - most of the AIDS research scientists were so concerned that they asked us not to use their names in this book. (Again, we thank those who allowed us to quote them.)

Everything from informed concern to uninformed panic is affecting work production. Public and private AIDS educational programs are diverting time and money from other programs. Owners and employees are devoting on-the-job and off-the-job time and energy to mulling over and worrying about AIDS. The work loss because of AIDS is presently awesome. It will get worse.

Work productivity is being influenced in other far less obvious ways. One of the business plant owners to whom we spoke told us about not being able to sleep many nights since he discovered that one of his many employees had AIDS. "Some mornings I'm just so damned tired that I can't think right. I can't get it out of my mind. I don't have AIDS; I'm just obsessed by what's going to happen to my company's employees because of it."

Our economy will be hit by such presently hidden effects of AIDS. The worry and panic will reduce our family, business, and national productivity.

Other formerly hidden economic effects of AIDS are surfacing.

Nutrition and AIDS

Nutrition remedies claiming to "treat what ails you" are beginning to list AIDS as one of the many diseases for which a cure is promised. Megadoses of vitamin C and special diet products such as blue-green algae and herbal capsules are among the questionable products for which such claims are being made.

> It is estimated that one billion dollars will be spent in the U.S. this year on fraudulent AIDS therapies including questionable nutrition products.
>
> In truth, little is known about the role of nutrition in AIDS. Organizations in the U.S. and Canada are beginning to address the need for information on this topic.
>
> Acknowledging that poor nutrition can contribute to a worsening condition and a nutritionally adequate diet may optimize the health of HIV infected individuals, members of the Society for Nutrition Education resolved at their 1987 Annual Meeting "to urge Health and Welfare Canada and the U.S. Department of Health and Human Services to integrate nutrition education into their AIDS programs." (Canadian Public Health Association, 1987)[5]

"Fraudulent AIDS therapies" are beginning to erode some of our work results. Work savings are being thrown away on hopeless, futureless AIDS "cures." Even fake claims from unqualified "doctors" are occasionally being paid.

Charlatans offering "medical" treatments and/or "spiritual" help to both AIDS victims and AIDS victims' families and friends are emerging. The number of such fakes will increase, and they will prey on persons' emotional and physical vulnerability. They will present themselves as members of the helping professions: Counselors, medical doctors, scientists, and religious or holy men.

Every charlatan and every fraudulent therapy for AIDS victims reduces saved work earnings, thus reducing present and future economic growth. All the saved capital that resulted from work is thrown away and unavailable for investment growth.

ALL BUDGETS ARE LIMITED: YOURS, BUSINESSES' & GOVERNMENT'S

Surface examples of some AIDS related work efforts will illustrate just how much work is being expended to deal with AIDS. Presently, a lot of money is being spent on AIDS research, AIDS education, and AIDS treatment. Expenditures on AIDS are already hitting your family, business, and national budgets.

The two most obvious AIDS costs that affect our budgets are public education and public health and social services. Since specific governmental expenditures go unnoticed by most of us, we do not pay attention to just how much is being spent on AIDS education and care.

Every educational campaign to inform people about AIDS affects work supply: The work necessary to develop the educational program; the work necessary to produce the materials for the educational program; the work necessary to disseminate the educational information, etc., all affect available work.

Furthermore, money which was earned through work is spent on all the supplies being used in all those phases of an educational campaign. Money only has value if that piece of paper represents something real, namely work.

We know that business and tax dollars are being spent on AIDS educational campaigns. Sometimes it is all so seemingly remote that we forget that every dollar spent on AIDS education cannot be spent anywhere else. Since anyone's budget - yours, businesses', government's - is always limited, if we spend money in one area, that money cannot be spent in another area.

We could not find comprehensive dollar numbers for the cost of AIDS education in the United States, but the money is being spent. The federal government has initiated its AIDS education campaign. Furthermore, "The number of states mandating AIDS education in public schools has tripled in the past six months, with 17 states and the District of Columbia now requiring such instruction, the National Association of State Boards of Education said Thursday." (Connell, 1987)[6]

One small example gives us some idea about AIDS educational costs: "For $19,000, a Charlottesville, Va., cartoonist (Charles Thompson) produced a 22-minute cartoon video on AIDS for school use. The revenue so far for Mr. Thompson and his distributor: About $750,000. With more than 5,000 copies sold, the film has outperformed Mr. Thompson's herpes blockbuster and become the cartoonist's biggest success in 15 years of making educational films." (Roger Ricklefs, 1987)[7]

We are certainly not knocking Mr. Thompson's product nor his success. AIDS education is much needed. Our point has to do with AIDS educational costs. Mr. Thompson's $750,000 is compensation for his work, apparently reasonable compensation, because schools are paying for his work. But $750,000 is a drop in the bucket when we consider federal and state AIDS educational costs.

Since no magic fairy godmother exists to cover AIDS educational costs, citizens must cover those costs. Those costs are coming out of our individual family budget through taxation. Your family budget and all other family budgets that include taxes are footing the AIDS education bill. So are businesses.

At the same time, all tax paying families and businesses are also supporting AIDS care costs, partially or wholly, directly or indirectly.

AIDS COSTS

Everyone producing work is in some way supporting AIDS care costs. We are supporting AIDS care costs in these ways:

1. Drug companies are investing money in their research and development programs to discover diagnostic procedures, safety and treatment procedures, and effective drug therapies for AIDS. They must support their costly research and development programs. Research and development requires enormous amounts of money.

   Until a product is produced, tested, and approved, it is all cash outflow; all cost/no profit. To support their research and development programs, drug companies pass the cost on to consumers buying the drug company's other products. A drug company's AIDS research and development costs can come out of our family budgets through other products we buy. Everything from camera film and shampoo to our prescription drug purchases can contain drug companies' AIDS research and development costs.

If the drug companies did not pass research and development costs along to consumers, no drug companies would exist very long if they tried to develop new products. They, too, have to break even or make a profit if they are going to survive. They are just as limited as our family budget.

2. All for-profit hospitals encounter losses because patients do not pay. The same is true for doctors. Corporations and individual doctors have to cover their losses and overhead the same as everyone else. AIDS losses are being passed to us through our increased bills, which we will discuss in more detail later.

3. All types of businesses are affected by AIDS costs. Costs for employee assistance programs are increasing. Employee assistance programs are educating employees about AIDS and dealing with AIDS worker cases. Employee assistance programs and employers are also spending time/work dealing with the real and possible decreased efficiency of employees working alongside AIDS carriers - fear can do more than lead to learning; fear can also immobilize and/or lead to panic acted out in the work place.

Employer share of medical insurance costs are and will continue to increase due to AIDS case costs. Disability costs are and will continue to increase because of increasing AIDS disability cases.

AIDS related costs to business are increasing the costs of all sorts of products and services. Whether or not your company employs an AIDS victim, your company is presently being affected. Other companies supplying your company with goods and services have been affected. Their overhead has increased due to AIDS related costs. That increases the costs to your company.

All other companies from whom you buy anything and everything are experiencing the same flow through of costs. Eventually, these increasing costs land in the budget of the final consumer, the family budget. As AIDS cases increase, price increases will progressively become greater. Those price increases will end up in all our family budgets. All costs eventually end up in workers' - our source of work - budgets.

4. Insurance costs are being affected by AIDS claims, which we will discuss in detail later. That affects, directly or indirectly, all earned family budgets.

5. Governmental expenditure on AIDS is already astounding. Three quotes provide the case:

> "A special $30-million emergency fund has been established to help low-income AIDS patients purchase the expensive drug AZT, health officials said Friday." (Washington (UPI), 1987)[8]

> "Surgeon General C. Everett Koop estimated Friday it could cost Americans as much as $16 billion by 1991 to cope with AIDS, which he called the [sic] 'the most vicious of infectious diseases in the history of the race.' " (Journal Wires, November 7, 1987)[9]

> "Driving the urge to a more comprehensive strategy against AIDS are ever more frightening projections of the cost of the disease. It is now estimated that AIDS will cost the nation $10 billion to $15 billion per year by 1991, not counting lost earnings and output. Patient care alone will cost $8 billion as the number of people diagnosed with the disease rises from the current 45,000 to about 270,000. If drugs are developed to stave off the disease among AIDS-virus carriers - who can remain uninfected for years - costs could rise even higher. By 1991, an estimated 5 million Americans will carry the virus. By 1992, medicaid costs are expected to jump 600 per cent, from $400 million now to about $2.4 billion. Taxpayers will foot the bills. (Steve Findlay, 1987)[10]

Every worker will share the burden of such costs. Every business will also share the burden of such costs. And those costs are presently trivial when we examine the future of the AIDS pandemic.

When AIDS researchers talk about the present AIDS situation just being the "tip of the iceberg," we rarely see data projecting the future situation. Dr. Browning projected the future AIDS deaths (see Table I).

If anyone thinks Dr. Browning's death figures are unreasonable and/or inflated, please offer that person these projections:

> Dr. Allan Salzberg, chief of medicine at the Veterans Administration Medical Center in Miles City, Montana ". . . proposed testing of sexually active people on a yearly basis, starting in their teens and continuing until about age 50. That approach would be the least discriminatory," he said.

> "Based on mathematical projections," Salzberg said, "this plan would lead in the year 2006 to 4.4 million people dead or sick from AIDS, 1.8 million carriers, and an average annual direct cost of $20 billion."

TABLE I

AIDS DEATHS

% AIDS DEATHS	DOUBLING TIME (MO)	DATE	NUMBER DEAD	U.S.
.013	21.8	1988	32,000	This assumes that about 10% of AIDS deaths are presently unreported; that the present rate of deaths will slow down (as per N-th-order (2nd) fit of present state death data can be projected), and that no cure will be found. ~ 50% of the population will survive.
.026	30.6	1990	64,000	
.052	44.7	1993	128,000	
.104	58.4	1997	256,000	
.208	58.9	2002	512,000	
.416	58.9	2007	1,024,000	
.832	58.9	2012	2,048,000	
1.664	58.9	2017	4,096,000	
3.328	58.9	2022	8,192,000	
6.656	59.4	2026	16,384,000	
13.312	75.1	2032	32,768,000	
26.624	89.2	2038	65,536,000	
53.248	98.0	2046	131,072,000	

by Dr. Browning

"With a do-nothing approach," Salzberg said, "these projections put the toll that year at 25 million sick or dead, 40 million carriers, and a direct cost of nearly $120 billion." (Associated Press, 1987)[11]

Whether we look at AIDS death and dying costs or lost productivity resulting from dying and dead workers, someone must "take up the economic slack." Unless we want to experience a severe decline in our standard of living, costs and lost productivity must somehow be covered. It will be workers, from manual laborers to top management, who have to cover the costs and make up for lost productivity.

Healthy citizens will have to support all the economic costs of AIDS. Work is the only thing that will keep our economy going.

AIDS VIRUS - THE ENEMY

Every sector of our economy will be progressively impacted by AIDS. That, of course, will affect all of our budgets. No American has ever seen anything, not even war costs, affect the economy as AIDS will.

The AIDS issue is like a national or world war issue. When we are being attacked, conservatives and liberals lay aside political issues and unite to confront the enemy. Survival issues take precedence over political issues.

**FIGURE 1
FUTURE AIDS DEATHS**

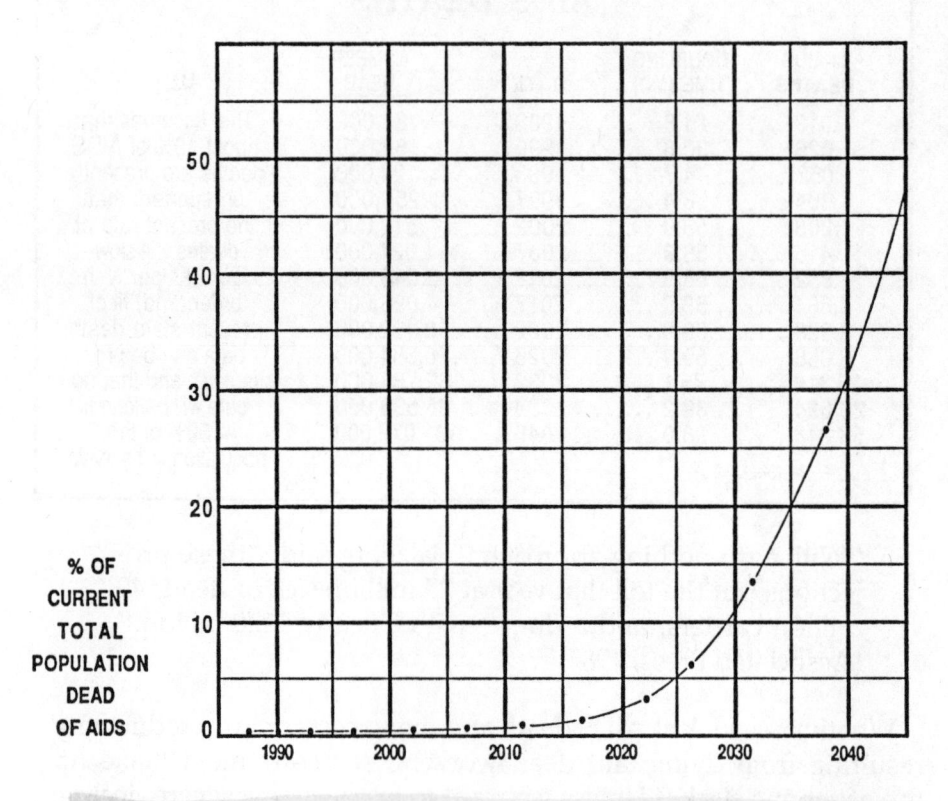

% OF CURRENT TOTAL POPULATION DEAD OF AIDS

(graph showing exponential curve rising from near 0 in 1990 to approximately 45% by 2040, with y-axis labeled 0, 10, 20, 30, 40, 50 and x-axis labeled 1990, 2000, 2010, 2020, 2030, 2040)

Although AIDS has become entangled in some political issues, AIDS is not a political issue. AIDS is a virus. AIDS is everyone's enemy. AIDS attacks human bodies and causes health, social, and economic chaos.

Even if a person never contracts AIDS, the virus can still devastate that person's life. Everyone has not died in a world war any more than everyone will die from AIDS. But anyone who lives beside the dying through a war is deeply affected. So it is with AIDS and AIDS will never ask for a cease fire.

Indeed, we have an enemy. But it is neither the homosexual nor drug using populations. Our enemy is not the people carrying the virus. Our enemy is the virulent mutating AIDS virus - the most rapidly mutating virus mankind has ever seen.

In assessing all the dangers, including the economic dangers, we need to remember what the enemy is. A clear, consistent focus on the enemy can lead us to wise decisions.

Panic will not lead to wise decisions and actions. Panic will lead us to further social atrocities and social upheaval. Prejudice and panic can lead to actions against all kinds of population or social groups who have no more connection to the AIDS pandemic than the Jews had to the Black Plague pandemic. Just as Dr. Browning described, groups can suffer the brunt of cruelty even though they have nothing to do with the cause of the panic.

We need to remember that everyone is involved in the analyses and decision making process concerning AIDS. All scientific, social, and economic situations and decisions will ultimately involve all of us. We all need to become knowledgeable concerning AIDS.

The longer people remain oblivious to the AIDS facts, the worse this pandemic will be. When you're on the front line, it doesn't help you to deny the artillery!

AFRICAN AIDS:
Mirror for Our Future AIDS

The spread of AIDS in Africa is ahead of the spread in the United States:

> The high-risk-states where the male-to-female ratio of victims is evening out show that the United States is following the AIDS pattern set by Africa. There, it is largely a heterosexual disease. Africa is about five years ahead of the rest of the world in its epidemic, the CIA notes. (Jack Anderson and Dale Van Atta, 1988)[12]

As you examine the available data*, we recommend that you look at African as well as United States information. The present situation in many African countries can alert us to future dangers to our lives and livelihoods.

Some brief descriptions of the present African situation indicate the severity of the impact of AIDS on many African countries.

---

*Sapiens Press will begin publishing *World AIDS: The Newsletter* in July, 1988. Aaron and Browning will be contributors. If you would like a comprehensive monthly information source concerning AIDS worldwide, we recommend such a monthly summary source.

It is difficult to say what the final toll will be. Regardless of its size, however, much of it will be felt in Africa. In some African countries epidemiological results show that a sizable fraction of people in the sexually active age groups are already infected. The high prevalence of infection in Africa is due partly to the fact that universal testing of the blood supply is beyond the economic reach of most African countries. As a result, the virus is still being transmitted by contaminated blood. In addition, it appears that the virus has had more time to spread in Africa than it has in any other part of the world. (Gallo, 1987)[13]

Because homosexuality is relatively rare in Africa, AIDS there is transmitted overwhelmingly by heterosexual contact. Men and women are equally affected by the epidemic. (Klingholz, 1987)[14]

The highest rates of infection are invariably in African prostitutes, with figures ranging from 27 to 88 per cent. More alarming are the figures of 10–20 per cent from blood donors and antenatal clinics, as these are not high-risk groups in Western terms. (Newmark, 1986)[15]

A personal interview we had with a nursing nun extends our picture of AIDS in Africa. She was a nursing nun for 35 years and also ran a medical mission. Author interview with Sister Jerome from Zambia:

> AIDS is on the rampage in Africa. Reports are that the bigger hospitals in Zambia show ten out of twelve blood tests AIDS positive.
>
> The government first ignored AIDS. Now it has established special clinics for educating people concerning the AIDS threat. However, it is a terrible educational problem.
>
> Ours is a very promiscuous society. The women are so poor that they sell themselves for money. And many of them are ignorant and don't understand disease transmission. Educating is a real problem, particularly when eating is a primary issue with the uninformed.
>
> Doctors, nurses, everyone in the health field is very much concerned. The Ministry of Health holds seminars for us and emphasizes self-protection against AIDS.

In the bush we always wear gloves when we deliver babies. We don't give many blood tests in the bush, but when we do, we also wear gloves.

Health professionals in Zambia know that we must take AIDS very seriously. We see the results - the "slims" or "skinnys," we call it. We see people just waste away. The government now makes sure we're all informed. No one ignores or minimizes in Zambia anymore.

The Ministry of Health informed us at a professional seminar recently that Zambia's population of 5,000,000 will decline to 2,000,000 by the year 2000 if things continue as they're going now.

Right now, once you've got it, you've just got it. There's no hope. And it's also a signal that there's no hope for the people around you. One person with AIDS indicates that many others in that person's village also have AIDS.

When we diagnose a person as having AIDS, we just have to send him home to die. That's the most humane thing we can do.

There's nothing our hospitals could do other than very temporarily prolong a miserable life. The hospitals simply can't afford to extend doomed lives. We have trouble enough just helping other patients who could live and thrive if they get some medical care.

We just have to send AIDS patients home to their villages to die. (Sister Jerome, December, 1987)

IMPACT OF AIDS ON THE FAMILY ECONOMY

While we face many very similar problems with AIDS, African AIDS related problems are also different from the United States situation. The United States is a far wealthier nation. We are far more industrialized/mechanized than Africa. And we have more modern resources available to us. Our population also differs significantly from African families. U.S. citizens are better educated than Africans. Our overall standard of living is higher. We marry later, and more women are working in the U.S. who earn far more than African women. We live longer; 12.1% of our population is 65 or older (1986 U.S. survey), which is a much higher elderly population than found in Africa.

Lack of Supportive Families

That all seems to bode well for us, at least on the surface. However, some of our population characteristics indicate that we may face some even greater problems than Africa in the near future. For example, Sister Jerome said, "We just have to send AIDS patients home to their villages to die." Because of evolving United States family characteristics, we may not have enough "villages."

"Villages" really represents available people - by far, most often family members - who will care for the AIDS victims while they are dying. In the U.S. the extended family has to a great extent disappeared.

Although African AIDS costs will never be the same as United States AIDS costs because the U.S. does not send all or most of its AIDS victims "home to die," African AIDS costs are obviously mounting. Furthermore, African countries do not have the economic resources to deal any differently with AIDS.

> "The prospects of routine testing [for AIDS] seem poor without the help of foreign aid. To put the overall financial problem even more starkly," according to Quinn et al., "the cost of caring for ten AIDS patients in the United States (approximately $450,000) is greater than the entire budget of a large hospital in Zaire, where up to 25 per cent of the pediatric and adult hospital admissions have HIV infection." (Newmark, 1986; Quinn, 1986)[16]

As that quote further indicates, the United States is and will be facing mounting demands for foreign aid requests for AIDS costs from African countries. We are faced with supporting AIDS costs in the United States while we also contribute financial support to those costs in foreign countries. Unless African countries receive Western economic help, they have little chance.

> Even if an effective vaccine against AIDS becomes available in a few years, no one in Africa will be able to afford it. In the same region where mankind took its first steps more than four million years ago - in Ethiopia, Kenya, Uganda,

Zaire and Tanzania - *Homo sapiens* is now in danger of being wiped out. (Klingholz, 1987)[14]

The African AIDS predicament also portends what the United States work force will face (I. S. Okware, Ministry of Health in Entebe, Uganda): A total of 1,138 cases of AIDS have been reported in Uganda, Okware says, about 85% of which occur among the sexually most active age group - men and women in equal numbers between 15 and 40 years of age. These include some of Uganda's most productive adults, in professional and economic terms, and Okware predicts that the impact of AIDS-related deaths among this group could be devastating to the country's welfare. (From the Third International Conference on AIDS, Washington, D.C., Barnes, 1987)[17]

We, too, will be faced with having our most productive adults sick and dying of AIDS. Our sexually active age group in the United States will face serious decline if macho(a) philandering does not stop. Naturally, such a population loss will affect our overall work force and economy.

No doubt exists that AIDS will profoundly affect every aspect of our economy. Work that supports all of us will become decreasingly available while the need for work to support those dying of AIDS and already dead will substantially increase. We will have increasing demands for work but inadequate supplies of work.

OUR BASIC ECONOMIC ASSUMPTIONS
All Economies Are Limited

All economies - family, business, government - are limited. Supply is limited. Demand is limited. Whether we look at the ancient elements of earth (air, fire, and water), or examine labor (productivity and efficiency), we discover that everything and anything is limited on Earth.

Working People = Work = People's Supply

In a family, the economy is usually determined by pay-for-work. If one person works and the other stays home, the monetary supply is determined by the working person's pay. If two family members work, that determines the monetary supply.

The family economy can be influenced by other work. In families that repair and make their clothes, repair their cars and houses, or build additions to their homes, "value-added" also goes into the family economy. Nonetheless, the supply was created through work - it just did not get taxed.

Outside influences such as lotteries and inheritances can affect the family monetary supply. However, those are anomalies. In the course of most persons' lives, those are irregularities. We need to remember that, in the first place, someone(s) had to make (earn/create) that monetary supply for anyone else to get it.

The same is true for the family economy that comes from government welfare and/or charity. Someone(s) always has to make (earn/create) the supply before it can be given to anyone else. And it does not matter what form the supply takes. It can be wealth in the form of gathered sea shells in a primitive society or $1,000,000,000 in cast gold. No matter - someone had to expend the energy to create the supply.

The same is true for business. After the initial capital investment (which is analogous to our parents' investment of work/supply during childhood), a business economy is determined by work. No business has a supply of anything without work.

It does not matter whether the supply is tangible or not. Information service firms must expend the energy to gain saleable knowledge. A physician with twelve years of informational training has a supply. A management consultant with twelve years of informational training has a supply. Both have a particular supply to provide that consumers will buy.

Any business economy is usually determined by pay-for-work. No supply/no work; no work/no supply. The amount of work, not the amount of time worked, (efficiency) determines the supply.

Just as the family economy, the business economy can be influenced by outside forces. But any influx of supply must come from a source that already made (earned/created) that supply. Business supplies, as family supplies, are created from work.

Much to many people's initial amazement, a government economy is determined by pay-for-work. [No, this is not a joke.] First, no government would have any monetary supply if its citizens did not provide that supply. The citizens must provide the governmental supply from what they have made (earned/created) . . . their supply. Second, the government's very existence is dependent upon its own supply. For example, in the United States the government guarantees these things for its citizens: "Life, liberty, and the pursuit of happiness."

The government's pay for work - its own supply - must come from its own work in supplying "Life, liberty, and the pursuit of happiness" for all its citizens. Like the doctor or management consultant who supplies intangible information and benefits, the government must also make (earn/create) its supply.

In the United States if the government does not supply what it has guaranteed, it will cease to exist by popular demand and highest law. U.S. citizens are obligated in their Declaration of Independence "to throw off such government, and to provide new Guards for their future security" if their government does not perform its proper functions.

Work = Supply

Sometimes truly unusual situations distort our economic vision. Individuals, businesses, and governments occasionally hit a "strike." They "strike" oil or gold, and the work = supply theory seems to go out the window. But we need to examine that.

In cases where minerals are discovered, it is true that individuals, businesses, and governments may not work many hours nor work very efficiently. However, oil provides work directly: Refined oil will run factories and cars and provide energy more efficiently than any number of men or man work hours could. Gold provides work indirectly. Gold buys oil, gas, or electricity that in turn provides work energy.

Natural resources are limited. The energy natural resources supply is limited. (We saw what can happen with limited natural resources when oil prices doubled.)

Individuals, businesses, and governments that inherit money, win lotteries, or strike oil or gold have no supply left when the original direct or indirect work results are gone. Then, they are no different than the family members who work to have a supply of anything. Those who have used up their "work" resources will have to find their own "work" if they want supply of anything.

The instances where work = supply does not seem to apply are these:

1. When someone else's work ends up providing supply to a nonworking person or entity. That happens with gambling winnings, inheritances, welfare payments and supports of all types, charitable contributions, and even pay to civil "servants" who are not working.

2. When a natural resource strike is made, and the natural energy from that resource strike directly or indirectly supplies the work or the natural resource buys the work.

In both of those instances, either a natural resource directly or indirectly provided the work or other people furnished the work. In any case,

WORK = SUPPLY

NO WORK = NO SUPPLY sooner or later

ALL ECONOMIES ARE LIMITED.

Work = Supply explains why we now have more of all material things than at any other time in history. Oil, gas, and other natural resources can produce work. Today computers and robots can provide the work. By using natural resources and machines, we have more of everything today. Yet we work far fewer hours: "In the U.S., the decline was from about 60 hours per week in 1870 to less than 40 hours at present." (Simon, 1985)[18]

No Work = No Supply, sooner or later.

It should be noted at this point that machines have not been created that invent themselves, build themselves, and run themselves. Machines are invented, built, and run through people's work. Machines do not eliminate people's work. People's types of work and job descriptions change because of the machines people invent. Through machines, people also increase their own and other persons' efficiency.

Unlike some natural resources, machines do not innately have energy that will produce work. However, neither natural resources nor machines produce energy/work that can be used by mankind without man's harnessing natural energy/work or inventing and building the machines that perform the work. Even if the energy/work exists and is moving powerfully as in a raging river, the energy/work simply moves on without man's intervention.

By capturing and utilizing natural resources and inventing and building machines, modern man has enormously increased his own work efficiency. More work is produced today than at any other time in history because man has harnessed natural resources and put

Mother Nature to work through the machines that man has invented and built.

Our greatly increased work efficiency does not change the facts. Working people are necessary to produce the work/energy that provides people's supply.

WORKING PEOPLE = WORK = PEOPLE'S SUPPLY

Even those who "live off the land" also have to expend the energy/work to gather the bounty.

You may want to remember these fundamental hypotheses and test our assumptions:

WORKING PEOPLE = WORK = PEOPLE'S SUPPLY

WORK = SUPPLY

NO WORK = NO SUPPLY, sooner or later

ALL ECONOMIES ARE LIMITED

What Klein calls dynamic "phenomenological laws (i.e., seeing is believing)" can be used to test each of our business/economic predictions. (Klein, 1984)[19] With the passage of future months, you will begin to see the impact of AIDS on U.S. business and our economy.

No matter what economic level we examine, we are always ultimately led back to individual workers and family budgets. Everything that influences business and government economies ultimately affects the budgets of those producing the work. Since the overall cost of AIDS is growing, we will progressively see AIDS' direct impact on family budgets.

As just a few years pass, the impact of AIDS on the U.S. and other countries will become unavoidably obvious. Businesses and economies throughout the world will be hit by the AIDS pandemic. Now and as this pandemic unfolds, please use the phenomenologically obvious and test our analyses in your own mind.

Two major things have happened to American families: (1) People have moved away from their original homes - parents and children alike - and family members do not see one another very often; (2) more women are working and returning to work sooner after births than any time in our history. (*American Demographics,* quoted in *The Wall Street Journal,* February 4, 1988, p. 23)

Moving Families

All studies on bonding and attachments that we have ever read clearly point to the necessity of human interaction for bonding and attachment to occur and continue. Many Americans hardly ever see their grandparents, let alone their cousins, etc. With parents and children moving not only frequently but also long distances from one another, their bonds and feelings of attachment are damaged.

> One in five people - about 45 million of us - moved in 1984–85 according to Census Bureau figures released in late December. That was an increase of 7.1 million moves over the year before, and it was the largest total since the bureau started collecting that information in 1948.
>
> About 30 million of those people moved to homes within the same county. About half of the rest changed from one county to another within the same state, and the rest moved from one state to another. (*Stone Company Newsletter*, 1988)[20]

Family separations and movements over long distances naturally weaken parent/child and nuclear family/extended family ties. Without on-going contact, familial bonding and attachment generally erode over time. Even in the initially very emotionally close families, if the family members are separated for long periods of time, the best intent does not make up for the loss of contact.

Working Women

The problem of long distances between family members is made even worse by the reality of working women. Women have been principally responsible for scheduling and maintaining social interaction in the U.S. When an American woman works, she normally has designated, scheduled, limited vacation time.

Working women with families already have "exhaustively difficult" lives. (Beck, 1987)[21] Their constantly compressed schedules simply do not allow for a lot of time to encourage family interactions, particularly over long distances [as one of the authors knows full well].

That brings us to another huge difference between African and U.S. populations. In African countries as many women work as in the United States, but their work is often quite different. The African women who till the fields, make articles by hand, etc., are in a much different social situation than American women who work in offices, restaurants, hospitals, etc.

American women work in an industrialized society. African women work in a mixed industrialized-agrarian society. In rural African villages, a woman can strap a child - her own or an AIDS victim's - on her back and go to the field. Handmade articles can be made in village homes while an African woman cares for a dying AIDS victim.

The vast majority of American women working for wages would get fired if they attempted to take children to work on a consistent basis. And most Americans don't have the opportunity to "take their jobs home." An industrial society simply works differently than an industrialized-agrarian society.

By and large, American women will not be available to care for AIDS victims and/or their survivors. Instead, AIDS will force more women into the work force. As U.S. productivity decreases due to AIDS deaths and economic demands to support the dependent, dying, and dead increase, the pool of presently unemployed women will be progressively compelled to help support the social costs.

Breakup of Nuclear Families

And the story gets worse. Not only extended families but also nuclear families have broken up and no longer exist. With about half of our population getting divorced, the United States has numerous single parent families.

Ex-wives will not support ex-husbands who are dying of AIDS, and ex-husbands will not support ex-wives who are dying of AIDS. With many Americans losing both the extended family situation and the nuclear family love and support system, the economic burden will fall on the rest of society.

Burying The Dead

The U.S. economy will have to support probably the majority of dying AIDS victims. We will have to bury the dead AIDS victims, something not to be ignored.

High Cost of Dying of AIDS

Funeral directors in some cities are charging $250 to $800 extra for handling the bodies of AIDS victims. Accused of gouging, the directors explain that they often must hire outside embalmers and other additional personnel to prepare the AIDS bodies. They also point out that, after working on the bodies, they must disinfect their labs and throw away gloves and other items that may be contaminated.

In some states, funeral directors are permitted a surcharge for handling victims of hepatitis, leprosy, tuberculosis, rabies, cholera and some 45 other communicable diseases. Jim Allen, executive officer of the California Board of Funeral Directors and Embalmers, explains: "The state generally permits funeral directors to pass on to the public the cost of their taking special precautions." (*Parade Magazine*, June 28, 1987, p. 16)

After burying the AIDS victims, American families will be faced with the overwhelming burden of supporting the AIDS victims' survivors: Husbands or wives, children, and/or boyfriends or girlfriends who are also dying of AIDS. The AIDS-free orphans who survive their AIDS parents will also be supported by us.

No Home For Many

Many Americans do not have a "village" to go home to while they are dying. And many of the Americans who would have a home to go to if they were dying of cancer will not find a "welcome home" from even their parents. AIDS in the United States provokes enormous fear, shame, guilt. Many parents simply will not allow their children who are dying of AIDS to come home.

At Fire Island in New York, realtors report exceptional buys for housing. The reason: Many male homosexuals have owned houses at Fire Island. As those AIDS victims die and their families inherit the victims' houses, some of the inheriting families will not even inspect the houses they have inherited. AIDS victims' houses have been sold without any of the victims' personal belongings being removed. Everything from clothing to the person's toothbrush is sold with the house.

Family members and friends have completely ostracized AIDS victims in many instances. And most of those AIDS victims have neither the personal resources left to support themselves nor a "village" in which they can die. United States citizens must support them.

SUBTLE BUT VERY REAL IMPACTS OF AIDS

The more in-depth we consider the consequences of AIDS on American families, the more profoundly we see a future economic disaster. AIDS is already beginning to hit American families in subtle ways that have not even been discussed until now.

Education and Art

Educational television will have fewer and fewer nature films from Africa. As African AIDS victims increasingly die and American AIDS victims progressively die in greater numbers, funds for African nature films - or most any nature films - will not be available. Support money for nature preserves will also be unavailable.

During an economic crisis, one of the first expenditure items that is reduced is entertainment, including educational entertainment. *ARTnews* provides us with a telling description of the present day situation:

> Foundations have played a big role in funding museums, but with the current economic crunch, more pressing charities (such as aid to the handicapped) are making greater demands on them. Corporate giving practices have changed, too. . . .
>
> On a national average, 55 per cent of those who work in museums are volunteers. It is wonderful that so many people believe enough in museums to give of their time to support them. Still, volunteers can be ephemeral. (Noble, 1988)[23]

Entertainment will change as sexual mores change, as will education. But other "fallout" effects will be less apparent. Public education and television programming will change, not just due to changes in sexual permissiveness, but also because of lack of funding.

Less of Everything

As more retiree-aged people and women are pressed into the work force by growing AIDS economic demands, fewer volunteers will be available. People will not be hired to replace the volunteers because the excess funds will not be available either. Lack of working people - for pay or not - and lack of money will affect all American families.

Fewer lakes and streams will be stocked with fish. Cities will pick up garbage less frequently. Less weed and litter control will be seen. Tax supported services of all kinds will decline.

Charitable organizations will suffer because disposable income will not be available from American families. Nationally and internationally, the needy will become progressively more needy. Research and development efforts in practically all areas will be cut back.

And all of this scenario is not scheduled for the distant future. It has begun:

> As it is, a disproportionate number of local [San Francisco] AIDS cases have been able to remain at home - and out of hospitals - because of agencies . . . that use a large number of volunteers to provide services to ailing patients. . . . hundreds of patients will continue to depend on community groups that are finding that they already need a steadily increasing number of volunteers.
>
> So far, most of the AIDS volunteers have been from the homosexual community, but this may well prove to be a shrinking base as more gay men themselves fall ill or are left to tend their own ailing friends and lovers. Although lesbians and heterosexual men and women are volunteering for AIDS work, their numbers are not great enough to come near to handling the work that needs to be done.

Measure of Humanity

> Local health officials need look no farther than New York City to see how mounting AIDS cases can cripple a health care system left unprepared for the epidemic. (Shilts, 1987)[24]

As AIDS progresses, our supply of volunteers will be depleted by:

- Declining numbers of people in our most productive age group;

- Younger people entering the work force;
- Older people returning to the work force to make up for lost productivity.

All types of low pay or no pay educational and artistic enterprises will suffer, as will American families. Some of those losses will cost us dearly, both immediately and long term:

> Nothing should count higher in a society than the care of its children, yet in the United States children have become a neglected constituency, comprising 40 per cent of the poor. Head Start, one of the jewels of the Great Society, has proven that high-quality early childhood education for the disadvantaged produces youngsters much more likely to finish high school, hold a job, and avoid welfare and crime. (*The New York Times*, 1987)[25]

The many longitudinal studies of Head Start children agree:

1. While in school they have less delinquency, truancy, and grade failure than those children who did not attend Head Start.

2. Head Start children also receive better grades and are "much more likely to finish high school, hold a job and avoid welfare and crime" than those children who did not attend Head Start.

Head Start is one of the best investment opportunities that the United States has now or for our future. But where can the funding come from if much of our income is spent on AIDS victims? With proportionally decreasing productivity, the money will not be available if our social and welfare costs increase substantially.

Back to "All Goods and Services Require Work" and "No Work = No Supply, sooner or later": Most of the work in the United States comes from families. The "Goods and Services" that American families can supply are limited by the amount of work they can perform. In short, we will only have just so much "goods and services" work products to spread around to everything.

We are all facing truly painful choices, but we need to begin making those choices now. Delay with our decisions will put us exactly where over-spending families end up: Choiceless or, if allowed to continue, bankrupt.

OUR PRESENT ECONOMIC SITUATION
(Some Say It Is Better; We Do Not Agree)

Studies concerning the economics of Americans need to be read carefully. Over time much has changed in the American family economy:

> The average American lives better now than 30 years ago and has to work fewer hours to pay for standard items like stoves, car tune-ups, haircuts and beer, according to an article in the September 14 FORTUNE magazine.
>
> . . . FORTUNE says every group of American - including the poor, the middle class, baby boomers, the elderly, blacks and women - are faring better today.
>
> The average American has twice as much buying power as in 1952, the magazine said. Income before taxes rose about 50 per cent from 1960 to $29,458 in 1986. And with two incomes and fewer children to support, the average family is better off. . . . (Associated Press, August 30, 1987, p. D7)[26]

To evaluate what "better" means, we need to examine what is being said in that article. In the 1950's far fewer women worked. Do two car families "fare better" when the second car is probably a necessity for getting to work?" Does the material possession of a second car = "better"?

We have far more two income families than during the 1950's. While we may have more spendable income, all the extra income requires work/time. That time/work requirement affects the entire family.

> "Changes in family structure have made it much more difficult to nurture children today," he (Bob Keeshan, better known as Captain Kangaroo) said. "It's a tough world for parents as well as for children because parents have much less time to give to children. We've had a hard day at the office and this little kid is trying to tell us about some little experience she's had that day. It's enormously important to her, but it couldn't be less important to us in our frazzled state, so we send her to watch television, and that goes on night after night."
>
> " 'The Captain' or 'Mister Rogers' or 'Sesame Street' can be

an auxiliary force, but they'll never be prime sources for nurturing a child or educating a child." (Clark, 1987)[27]

The entire family structure is affected when both husband and wife work. The traditional work role separations of the 1950's are continuing to break down. More men engage in child care, cooking, and all other types of household chores than previously. More women are involved in what were formerly male work roles.

In families with children, parents are more "frazzled" when both parents work. Less time is available - "quality" or "less quality" time. That affects many children in two income families.

"More is better." More of what? "Better" depends on a person's and family's definition of *better*.

Family Purchasing Power

We also need to examine whether or not we even have more real income to spend on material things. Based on 1977 dollars, our average weekly earnings in 1987 were $171 for private, non-agricultural work, per person. However, in 1979 our average weekly earnings for private, non-agricultural work, per person were $183. Inflation outstripped earnings. (Rostvold, 1988)[28]

American families are losing purchasing power. Our work-earned dollar simply buys less and less.

A *USA Today* story indicates what is really going on with American work-earned incomes.

> Our houses cost more than twice as much as they did a decade ago, but the USA's growing number of two-income families is helping keep up with the costs.
>
> The price of a home today is 116 per cent more than in 1977 - compared to an 87.6 per cent hike in the consumer price index over the same period.
>
> Among the League's (U.S. League of Savings Institutions) findings: 54.5 per cent of home-buying households now have two wage earners - up from 47.2 per cent in 1977.
>
> A greater number of first-time buyers select homes 25 years or older . . . and first-timers are more likely to buy condominiums - 16.3% vs. 11.9% for move-up buyers. (Landis and Guy, 1988)[29]

Socially dependent families and low income families are and will continue to lose economic ground. With the 1986 Tax Reform Act and limited United States liquidity, resources for charitable contributions and welfare payments will decline.

But it is not just no or low income families that are experiencing economic cutbacks:

> The stock market crash brought thousands of fast-track Wall Street careers to a screeching halt, inflicting burdensome financial and psychological damage on many in the army of laid-off investment bankers, traders and salespeople. (Cox, 1988)[30]

That American stock market crash hit everyone, directly or indirectly, upper income to no income families. "All Economies Are Limited." Any major influence on a major sector of our economy impacts all other sectors of our economy.

National Economy and Family Budgets

Our national economy is already in trouble. We are $2+ trillion in debt, and our national debt is growing. We have a $150 billion federal deficit for 1987. When that is coupled to our trade deficit, the 1987 American economy was $220+ billion short. The United States federal deficit for 1988 is projected to be $160 billion. All that means that Americans are facing a mini-crisis in our economy. (Rostvold, 1988)[30]

Everything that affects our national economy and our overall business economy influences American family budgets.

> Thus neo-classical theory has nothing to say about the shifting aggregate profitability of business. But - and I will not do the demonstrations - the Kalecki view does have something to say. In the Kalecki view gross capital income, or profits for short, under strict limiting assumptions, equals investment. Under looser assumptions, profits equals investment plus the government deficit; and under quite general conditions profits equals investment plus the government deficit plus the balance of trade surplus plus consumption financed by profit income minus savings financed by wage income. (From Minsky, 1980)[31]

These "Kalecki" equations reflect quite simple ideas such as that the workers who produce investment goods have to "eat." The output of consumer goods has to be allocated by price among the workers who produce consumer goods and those who produce investment goods. This implies that there will be an aggregate markup on labor costs in the sales proceeds of consumption producers equal to the wage bill in investment goods production. The Kalecki equations also reflect a well known phrase: Workers (in consumption goods production) cannot buy back what they produce.

The validation of business liability structures - i.e., the fulfillment of expectations about both the ability to meet payment commitments and the ability to refinance (fund or roll over) debts - depends upon current and expected profit flows. (Minsky, 1982; Kalecki, 1939)[32]

Ultimately, family, business, and government economies are inextricably related. The reason for that is simple: Any and all economies are based on work, and all work production comes from workers. No matter how much we influence productivity through mechanization, the foundation of all work production depends on individual workers.

As we lose workers to AIDS and have to support those dying of AIDS and their dependents, all support will eventually fall on our foundation: Individual workers and the American family. Each and every one of us will end up supporting AIDS costs, and that will severely lower our families' standards of living.

"There ain't no free lunch." Let's just hope that by the turn of the century we have something left to pay for family lunches.

INCREASING MEDICAL DEMANDS/ DECREASING MEDICAL PERSONNEL; INCREASING MEDICAL COSTS/ DECREASING ECONOMIC RESOURCES

The increasing costs for AIDS related research and development, social and welfare support, and medical care are apparent. Those costs are also compounding:

"Increased sophistication is needed in the application of social science within health promotion and increased facility in mobilizing cross-sectional resources to achieve public health objectives and generate confidence in approaching AIDS prevention." (Meyer, 1987)[33]

What may not be so immediately apparent is the real potential for a decrease in available medical personnel:

> FEAR OF AIDS could deepen a shortage of internists, researchers worry.
>
> A survey of 258 residents in internal medicine and pediatrics at seven New York teaching hospitals discovers that a quarter would prefer to avoid a career that involves treating AIDS patients. A fourth, if given a choice, would refuse to treat them. In the view of medical experts, this bodes ill for internal medicine, the primary-care specialty for AIDS and adults in general.
>
> The National Resident Matching Program says the number of residents in internal medicine already is at its lowest level since tracking began in 1978. It figures the country needs 2,000 more residents in the field. Now, with the AIDS fear, the National Association of Public Hospitals sees "a very real threat" that big urban medical centers will have trouble attracting and keeping the talent they need.
>
> SUCH HIGH-AIDS-INCIDENCE CITIES AS NEW YORK, SAN FRANCISCO, AND DALLAS COULD BE HARDEST HIT. [*The Wall Street Journal* emphasis][34]

Reasons exist for physicians and all medical personnel to be concerned about their personal contact with AIDS. In August 1987 *Nature* published this article by Charles M. Lent, Department of Biology, Utah State University:

AIDS: Another Threat

SIR - The public health threat from the AIDS (acquired immune deficiency syndrome) virus compels attention to laboratory practice. It appears[1] that blood from people with AIDS can infect others, either by intact mucosa or dermal cuts. These findings demand a review of many old, often comfortable, laboratory procedures. . . . we study the feeding behavior of medicinal leeches. . . . In feeding leeches, we routinely use human blood obtained from a hospital blood bank where it is tested for both AIDS and hepatitis virus, but all feeding experiments must now be conducted while wearing rubbers gloves, as AIDS is not always detected by the antibody test.

. . . All experiments in introductory physiology and biology courses that require students to be exposed to fresh blood, urine or saliva have now been cancelled (permanently, I suspect). (Lent, 1987; [1]III International Conference on AIDS)

Apparently, Dr. Lent was not over-reacting nor concerned too soon:

An unidentified lab worker has become infected with the AIDS virus, leading experts to call for renewed vigilance in safety procedures.

. . . More noteworthy, and perhaps more alarming, is that the lab worker suffered an "unapparent exposure," that is, no obvious major spill or needle-stick injury, prior to infection. . . . Scientists speculate the virus may have reached the worker's skin through an unapparent hole in gloves. (Chase, 1988)[36]

We need to add that the lab worker "infected was culturing concentrations of virus perhaps 1000 times higher than those found in the blood of an AIDS patient - thus raising risk exposure." (Chase, 1988)[36]

As we say here and have said elsewhere, informed medical workers, be they doctors, dentists, lab technicians, etc., are and should be quite concerned about AIDS. Medical personnel do not deal with normal populations. They deal with sick populations. Except for the atypical "yearly checkup visit," people are usually sick when they see medical people. That increases medical personnel's exposure to disease.

Of course, that also increases the likelihood of medical personnel contracting the very disease they are treating if the disease is communicable. Since AIDS is a viral disease, medical personnel treating AIDS patients simply increase their chances of contracting AIDS.

Everything discussed will increasingly reduce the availability of medical care for American families. "Baltimore's crusty sage, H. L. Mencken, grumbled, 'The true aim of medicine is not to make men virtuous. It is rather to safeguard and rescue them from the consequences of their vices.' " (Green, 1987)[37]

Medical personnel will increasingly become less enthusiastic about "safeguarding" and "rescuing" men from their vices. Increasingly, as the AIDS health dangers become more obvious, medical workers will leave the medical profession.

The AIDS related health dangers to medical doctors and hospitals are only part of the problem, however. Many costs to doctors and hospitals are dramatically rising. Medical equipment costs, including AIDS medical protection and treatment equipment, are significantly increasing. "AIDS Fears Alter Medical Products," everything from medical equipment to protective devices. (*The Wall Street Journal*, October 1, 1987)[38]

Doctors and hospitals have been sued for justified and unjustified reasons. The resulting legal costs and settlements have made malpractice insurance premiums skyrocket.

And that is not the end of the story. Dr. Miller describes other pertinent situations in the medical community:

> To my father, premature death was the constant enemy. Fifty years later I have been too successful at stalling death. I have prolonged the act of dying for poor souls whose times, by rights, had come. With the excuse of "saving lives," and with a little technology, I have justified tortures worthy of the Inquisition. The relatives of these patients have been twisted to the breaking point by the wonders of modern medicine.
>
> Protracted dying is an American epidemic. . . .
>
> Medical care, at its best, produces miracles at a bargain price. . . .
>
> But at its worst, modern medicine is wasteful and inhumane. We have not yet reckoned with the technology of dying; neither the cruelty nor the cost. Thus medical care is overpriced, and medical people are under attack.
>
> While I was at a medical conference, I overheard a group of physicians speak of serious matters. I realized that I had heard the same conversation a week before, 1000 miles away. Only the faces had changed.

Three of them no longer wanted to practice medicine. They looked to be in their early 50's. One had tried to discourage his son from applying to a medical school. They talked of bureaucratic hassles, senseless regulations, endless raises in insurance premiums. Their work was scanned by computers and picked apart by clerks. Four of them had been sued. (Miller, 1987)[39]

All doctors are to some extent being affected as that description from *Reader's Digest* indicates. Not only medical personnel's income is being threatened, but also their literal lives are at risk. We will see many more medical people leave their profession. As well, we will see increasing medical costs and decreasing medical services available to families.

Some families will be able to afford the costs. No matter what the costs, if the prevention, care, and/or treatment is/are effective, wealthy family members will figure out a way to get medical care and treatment. Most families do not have such economic resources available, however. Some families will receive inadequate medical care and treatment in the future. Poor families may receive little or no treatment in the future.

> Some health care facilities are already threatened.
>
> CHICAGO-Researchers on Thursday reported that already burdened public hospitals and major teaching institutions are caring for a disproportionate share of the country's AIDS patients.
>
> The problem will worsen unless such care - estimated to cost $8.5 billion by 1991 - can be restructured, the report by the National Association of Public Hospitals said.(Reuters, 1987)[40]

We need to remember that while all of our medical costs are escalating an unusually high number of people will be dying of AIDS. Those dying of AIDS will, again, most likely be in their most productive years. Healthy American families will be supporting everyone. When the economic pie is cut to serve everyone, less and less will be economically available to those healthy, working families.

We will have Art Myatt summarize for us as his words appeared in *The Humanist*, July/August 1987. (Myatt, 1987)[41]:

> *AIDS victims will make their demands on the same set of doctors and hospitals as everybody else. Directly or indirectly, we will all be affected by the epidemic.*

> *The general picture is that medical care will become both more expensive and of lower quality as the demand for it is greatly increased. This is absolutely elementary economics.*

AIDS IMPACT WILL NOT BE EQUAL

Major metropolitan areas will experience the most profound initial economic impacts of AIDS. Furthermore, specific minorities will increase their already disproportionate share of AIDS.

Major Metropolitan Areas Will Be Hit First

A study by Carliner and Bloom of the National Bureau of Economic Research indicates what we will be seeing in cities:

> . . . in New York, San Francisco and some other large cities where AIDS patients are concentrated, the economic impact "will be quite serious," said Carliner. . . .

> "If you live in a big city, you're going to feel it," he said. "It is going to show up in a variety of ways - lower housing prices, higher tax bills, disrupted insurance markets."

> Bloom said their study dealt only with New York and San Francisco because those cities now have the best statistics on the spread of AIDS. But he said eventually other cities, notably Los Angeles, Miami, Houston and Newark, N.J., also will feel the economic effects of the AIDS epidemic.

> The economists said that AIDS is spreading among intravenous drug users, a group that is less likely to have jobs and private insurance, and more likely to require public-supported medical care. Additionally, AIDS patients with jobs often will exhaust the limits of their health insurance

and are required to impoverish themselves before federal funds become available.

As a result, they said, AIDS patients as a group are more apt to depend upon tax supported health care than are patient groups with heart disease or cancer. (Associated Press, 1988)[42]

New York City is a good example of what we will be economically facing in the future in metropolitan areas:

> New York City is underestimating by half the projected cost of the spreading AIDS epidemic and is fiscally unprepared for its "terrible consequences," State Comptroller Edward V. Regan said yesterday.
>
> Mr. Regan said the state's Office of the Special Deputy Comptroller for New York City had estimated that AIDS would result in $2 billion in hospital costs in 1991 - at a cost to the city of $450 million - or twice as much as projected two months ago by the State Health Commissioner, Dr. David Axelrod.
>
> **Said Warnings were Rejected**
>
> "These are terrible figures," Mr. Regan said. "We think the public has a right to know about them and the city has to get itself prepared for the terrible consequences." But he said the city had repeatedly rejected his warnings that AIDS, acquired immune deficiency syndrome, "could require a significant increase in New York City spending."
>
> "It's obvious we're going to need more doctors, more money and more hospital beds," Dr. Joseph [City Health Commissioner] said. "The real question is will the Federal Government meet its responsibility to provide them."
>
> Dr. Joseph projects a cumulative number of AIDS patients of 40,000 by 1991. However, Mr. Regan said his estimates are three times higher, based on a projection that 6 per cent of the 450,000 infected people - or 27,000 people - will develop AIDS each year. (Sullivan, 1987)[43]

It is not just the inner cities that will be facing the problems of AIDS. Suburbs of metropolitan areas will also be seriously affected as AIDS leaps to those communities. "Just outside New York City, suburban doctors and social workers are struggling not only to treat their AIDS patients, but also to find places for them to live, buses to take them on errands, and neighborhoods to welcome them home."

> Schmitt goes on to describe the myriad of problems "straining" New York suburbs. " 'Suburban agencies are used to dealing with predominantly middle-class gay white men,' said Marge Eichler, an epidemiologist with the Connecticut Department of Health Services. 'Some agencies may feel uncomfortable dealing with IV drug users,' she said. 'It's a new group to them with an entirely different set of problems.' " (Schmitt, 1987)[44]

Formerly, as suburbs dealt primarily with "middle-class gay white men," the AIDS victims were paying for their own care. As more and more suburbs are forced to pick up the tab for the poor's AIDS care, suburbs will increasingly suffer. Even when agencies pool their resources as they are doing in Long Island, enough resources do not exist - not even now.

As AIDS patients leave the inner city and go home to suburbs, AIDs costs inevitably move to the suburbs. Suburbs simply are not equipped to handle the swelling AIDS population. Medical facilities, housing, transportation, and other support systems are not in place for AIDS victims in the suburbs.

Furthermore, social attitudes towards AIDS victims are not supportive. Unlike individuals with other diseases, parents and other family members often refuse to allow the AIDS victim to live with them. Private homes, nursing homes, and hospitals are refusing to become actively involved with AIDS care.

Suburbanites are refusing to increase their taxes to support AIDS victims. As one of our interviewees told us, "When AIDS victims are sick and dying in New York City or San Francisco, you don't have to see them. Those cities are so large that you can "hide" the AIDS people in some ghetto. Sure it affects people's taxes - when people find out just how much things may change. But for now, they just pay a little more in taxes and ignore the whole thing. But that's not true in the suburbs. If I asked my voters to raise taxes to support AIDS victims, I'd never hold public office again." (Elected Official, 1987)

The suburbs have just begun to deal with the AIDS problems. We are certain that the social and economic situations will only get worse in the suburbs.

Just as African AIDS cases can help us predict the coming world AIDS situation, metropolitan New York and San Francisco can help us detect what will happen in other major cities. If we use the models available, including the knowledge about the mistakes that have already been made, we can avoid some of the pitfalls of dealing with AIDS in other cities.

Some AIDS programs will cause a lot of turmoil. The National Academy of Sciences has recommended that sterile needles and syringes be made available to drug addicts, since needle sharing is "a known mode of transmission." However, such programs "go against the grain" of many Americans:

> But such programs have not been implemented anywhere in this country. The main reason appears to be politicians' reluctance to take any action that could be mistaken for tolerance of illegal drug use. In New York City, for example, former health commissioner Dr. David Sencer "periodically" proposed needle distribution to Mayor Edward Koch. He was rebuffed until August, 1985, five years into the AIDS epidemic, when Koch told Sencer, "If you don't mind being the fall guy, why don't you write a memo, and I'll circulate it." He did, and though for Sencer the proposal was "just epidemiological sense," the result was that "everybody said, Yeech," especially the district attorneys and police. Koch rejected needle distribution as an idea "whose time has not come and, based on the response, will never come." Recently, New York City's health commissioner, Dr. Stephen Joseph, finally proposed a small experimental program involving less than 1 per cent of the city's addict population. Despite the fact that AIDS has become the city's leading killer of young men and women, New York State rejected the plan last month, ostensibly because the experiment was scientifically unsound. . . . Meanwhile, the New York State Bar Association's Committee on Medicine and Law has urged the state to legalize the purchase of needles and syringes without a prescription. (Schwartz, 1987)[45]

The Atlantic ran a pertinent cover story on the City of Los Angeles in their January 1988 issue. Two articles in that issue foretell what the United States will encounter in many of its major cities:

> Aside from the enormous size of the local market, one rea-

son for Los Angeles's continued strength in manufacturing is its ability to combine First World managements, talent, and location with the Third World labor, provided by recent arrivals from Latin America and Asia. Without this plentiful cheap labor Los Angeles would lose much of its garment and furniture manufacturing and distribution industries to lower-cost locations. [p. 35]

The population of greater Los Angeles is also growing and diversifying. Now 12.6 million, the population is projected to reach 16.4 million by 2000 and 18.3 million by 2010. Greater Los Angeles, therefore, will retain in 2000 its current position as one of the twelve largest cities in the world, according to Peter Hall's *The World Cities*. This fact is impressive when it is considered in the context of urban growth around the globe. In 1950, Hall notes, seven of the world's twelve largest cities were North American or European. By 2000 only two - Los Angeles and New York - will be. Greater New York is not growing rapidly, but it will remain on the list because of its currently enormous population.

. . . the Los Angeles metropolitan area became the leading point of entry for legal immigrants to the United States. Since the late 1970's, moreover, Los Angeles has also gained hundreds of thousands of illegal immigrants.

As the metropolitan area's population increases, its ethnic composition is becoming less Anglo and more Latin and Asian. The Anglo population will drop from 60 per cent to approximately 40 per cent in 2010, while remaining stable in absolute terms, according to a recent report by Frank E. Hotchkiss, the director of regional strategic planning for the Southern California Association of Governments. The non-Hispanic black population will rise from 9 per cent to 10 per cent, increasing by approximately 800,000. The Asian population will grow from 6.2 per cent to 9.3 per cent, increasing by almost one million. The Hispanic population will rise from 24 per cent to 40 per cent, increasing by more than four million [pp. 41, 48]. (Lockwood and Leinberger, 1988)[46]

The Atlantic expands our scenario in their other story "Growing Pains." (Lemann, 1988)[47]

Los Angeles as a whole is preoccupied with two related issues right now: Immigration and development. In any objective comparison with other cities of its size, Los Angeles is blessed in both respects. Its immigrants fall generally into two groups: Illegal aliens from Mexico, who are very poor but aren't in a position to ask for much help from the government, and Asians, who are famous for being overachievers. It is very hard to make a case that immigrants are a drain on the city. But to understand politics in Los Angeles and what is likely to dominate the city's politics for the rest of the century, it is crucial not to underestimate how seriously these issues are taken. Ten years ago the movement for Proposition 13, which strictly limits property taxation, was often portrayed by the out-of-state press as another wacky California fad; now it looks like the truest harbinger of the national politics of the eighties. The interlocking issues of immigration and development, tempting as it may be to dismiss them, may well seem the same way ten years from now. [p. 58] (Lemann, 1988)[47]

Cities relying on "Third World Labor" or "cheap labor" of any kind have lower socio-economic population groups who are less educated. Due to lower socio-economic groups' lack of education, those groups are less likely to be aware of and informed about AIDS in general.

Thus far, education is our best prevention against the spread of AIDS. Yet billboards around Los Angeles advertise condoms for protection against AIDS. That only spreads AIDS if the uninformed continue to have nonmonogamous sexual relationships. Using condoms or not, sexual contact with multiple partners simply increases a person's likelihood of coming into contact with the AIDS virus. (Kaplan* 1987)[48]

Populations of urban areas tend to be more sexually permissive than rural populations. Urban populations also have higher incidence of drug abuse. Combine those characteristics with the lower educational levels of "cheap labor" and you have an AIDS time bomb.

---

*Kaplan's book, *The Real Truth About Women and Aids*, is as pertinent to men as it is to women. Anyone wishing to gain more information regarding sexual transmission of AIDS may want to read her book - unless that person is offended by extremely frank sexual discussions. Kaplan's book "pulls no punches." However, although Kaplan's information is accurate, Aaron finds the recommended "Dry Sex" practices more than a little dangerously challenging to aroused sex partners.

But there is another aspect to be addressed. On February 15, 1988, ABC News Radio reported that a Johns Hopkins study of work and taxation found as much as 1/3 of the world economy may be non-tax paying. In large cities, that "under-ground economy" is often part of the "cheap labor" that Lockwood and Leinberger discuss.

Lower socio-economic groups pay fewer taxes to begin with simply because they earn less. Furthermore, many of the "cheap labor" workers do not pay any taxes. A little taxes + no taxes = a need for a lot of social and welfare support.

American families will be faced with supporting the costs of low or no income AIDS victims. The United States will be forced to make enormously difficult choices: How much economic support can we afford for everything; how will the tax dollars be allocated?

Ultimately, all support requirements fall on American families and single individuals because they are the ones who supply the work.

Cities will be the first to experience the consequences of AIDS.

> More and more, AIDS is threatening to overwhelm inner-city people, who already endure enough hardship. Some say it is only a matter of time before the most important occupations at 8th and M [Washington, D.C.] - prostitution and drug dealing - are supplanted by the work of undertakers." (Wartzman, 1987)[49]

These are the U.S. cities reporting the most cases of AIDS, in descending proportions: New York, San Francisco, Los Angeles, Houston, Washington, D.C., Miami, Newark, Chicago, Philadelphia, and Dallas.

Without considering AIDS related health care costs, cities are already over-burdened by the problems of the homeless:

> McMurray-Avila [associate administrator of Health Care for the Homeless] agrees. "With health care for the homeless," she said, "the care is more important than the health sometimes."
>
> This is one trait that sets this clinic apart from others: Patients seek human contact as much as health care. Other differences are more apparent. Homeless clients often have to be asked to shower before they can be examined. Because of basic distrust of institutions or old habit, many won't use their real names and on return visits will use still another

pseudonym, making record-keeping virtually impossible. Need to track a patient down to give him or her the results of a test? First, guess which name to use. Then figure out how to find a person who lives on the street. Try telling a homeless person to take aspirin, drink plenty of fluids and rest - but *where?* (Engel, 1987)[50]

All larger cities are faced with similar problems. Street people without AIDS create huge economic burdens for cities. Now those street people are among the highest of the high-risk AIDS groups. As more street people contract and spread AIDS through either sexual contact or blood donations, cities will have to support the AIDS costs.

We may soon have taxpayers limiting property taxes and other forms of taxation through more universalized "Proposition 13s." Most everything indicates that Americans will say "no" to any more taxes. We are returning to a much firmer line of "no work, no pay" or support of any kind if a person is able to work.

So where will support for AIDS victims be found? Economic support from charitable organizations probably will not increase for AIDS victims. The 1986 Tax Reform Act knocked out so much of the tax deduction advantages for contributing to charity that charitable organizations are presently feeling that cut.

American families are not contributing to charity as they once did; neither are corporations. Such a stigma is attached to AIDS in general that AIDS anything is not a high priority for charitable contributions anyway.

Unlike the benefit concerts and other mass charity efforts for famine in Africa, AIDS - African or otherwise - will never gain such united mass charity support. Fears that Americans have for their own well being and their more universalized fears rule out the possibility of AIDS gaining a lot of social and economic support.

It will not be the states, either, that assume the economic support role for AIDS care. Just like cities, our states have their problems, too:

> Thirteen states (Florida, Illinois, Indiana, Iowa, Minnesota, Montana, Nebraska, New Mexico, North Dakota, Rhode Island, Tennessee, Wisconsin and Washington) now have subsidized risk pools for uninsurables. But they have to pay a high premium for their coverage, which many can't afford. (Quinn, 1987)[51]

States rely on exactly the same tax supporters as cities - good old tax paying, working Americans. We can all be certain that the economic prices for AIDS will land in each of our laps. That is why the AIDS virus is everyone's concern.

As we said previously, AIDS cases in cities and the economic impact of those AIDS cases on cities can be used to predict where we are headed nationally. Unless someone becomes a hermit - a non-tax paying hermit - he or she will experience the economic impact of AIDS. AIDS will spread from the cities to rural areas and hit all American families.

Specific Minorities Will Increase Their AIDS Proportions

We need to gain accurate information and develop on-going awareness about AIDS. Thus far, AIDS is very group(s) specific. It is not a widespread heterosexual disease - yet. Dunea in the *British Medical Journal* presents the United States AIDS details as of August 22, 1987:

> So far 90% of victims are drawn from two groups: The homosexuals - 2.5 million practising exclusively and 2.5 to 7.5 million practising intermittently - and the addicts, some 1.3 million. Only 4% have arisen through heterosexual contact, largely from sexual partners of addicts. Even among prostitutes spread is mainly by addicts, so that in Miami, for instance, 40% of inner city prostitutes but none from an escort service were found to be infected. About 2%, or 700 patients, are drawn from the 34 million who received blood transfusions before 1985, of whom 12,000 may have been exposed to AIDS. Another 1% comes from America's 20,000 haemophiliacs, of whom 70% are HIV positive and 330 have already developed AIDS. *Blacks and Hispanics* account for a disproportionate share of patients (11% and 8% of the population but 25% and 14% of patients with AIDS) and young blacks are five times more likely to develop the disease than whites. About 6% of cases have occurred in women, again mostly black (50%) or Hispanic (20%), often drug addicts (50%) or infected by sex with addicts (20%). (Dunea, 1987)[52]

It is obvious why homosexuals, addicts, and "haemophiliacs" have such high incidence of AIDS. They come into direct contact with the AIDS virus.

But why do "Blacks and Hispanics account for a disproportionate share of patients (11% and 8% of the population but 25% and 14% of patients with AIDS) and young blacks are five times more likely to develop the disease than whites?"

And even that is not the end of the story. Black and Hispanic proportions of the AIDS population are increasing. "The number of new AIDS cases among blacks and Hispanics reported to the Chicago Health Department in August exceeded that of whites for the third month this year, bringing to 47 per cent the minority share of new AIDS cases in the city in 1987." (Griffin and Galvan, 1987)[53]

So, again, what is happening? The answers are there if we piece them together.

First, "Researchers say the major difference in the incidence of AIDS between whites and minorities is the degree to which intravenous drug use and needle sharing is practiced within minority communities." (Schmidt, 1987)[54]

Second, we have the sexual mores of some blacks and Hispanics that significantly increase the likelihood of contact with the AIDS virus. Particularly in poor urban communities in which high incidence of intravenous drug use, needle sharing, and alcohol abuse occur, dangerous sexual contact is more likely to occur.

Drug and alcohol abuse lowers everyone's inhibitions, not just the sexual inhibitions of minority groups. But if more blacks and Hispanics are engaged in drug and alcohol abuse, they are also more likely to experience lowered social inhibitions and engage in risky sexual practices.

Far more unmarried teenage pregnancies occur among urban poor blacks and Hispanics than among the rest of the urban middle class population groups. That seems to indicate that premarital sex goes on, whether or not it is socially permissible.

Some experts have begun to talk about the disproportionate rates of AIDS among blacks and Hispanics:

> A health expert [Dr. Beny J. Primm] called Tuesday for special steps to curb the spread of AIDS among blacks, even if such steps are perceived as being racist.
>
> Although blacks are only 12 per cent of the U.S. population, they represent a quarter of all adult AIDS cases. . . .
>
> Blacks account for almost half of the women and 53 per cent of the children with AIDS, said Primm, executive direc-

tor of the Addiction Research and Treatment Corp. of New York. . . .

"I have, when necessary, actually cajoled and advised my colleagues who are white," said Primm, who is black. ". . . My friends are afraid they will be called racists if they cite these statistics. I have said it is better to be called a racist now than to be called a conspirator who was in a conspiracy of genocide 5 to 10 years from now when many, many more blacks will die because of your silence."

In certain high-risk neighborhoods, sex education could begin even at the pre-kindergarten level, Primm said. "The earlier we begin the better off we are," he explained. (Curry, 1987)[55]

Another community leader points to the existing situation:

Michael Lomax, the chairman of Atlanta's Fulton County Commission, said that the black establishment's difficulty in dealing with AIDS was part of a larger predicament. "It is a matter of coming to terms, at last, with the fact that there are problems within our community that were not imposed upon us by white society," he said.

"Intravenous drug use, teenage pregnancy and sexual promiscuity are behaviors that are pathological in our own community, and we must come to grips with that, to take responsibility." (Schmidt, 1987)[54]

The problems of Hispanic AIDS may be even more complicated than AIDS within the black urban populations:

Community health workers say the actual number of AIDS cases among Hispanics could be higher than official reports because many Hispanics hide the disease due to distrust of institutions, avoidance of doctors and taboos associated with homosexuality.

Hispanics who are illegal aliens are said to avoid reporting the disease because they fear deportation or having their amnesty requests rejected. (Griffin and Galvan, 1987)[53]

Despite the popular stereotype of the free-wheeling "Latin lover," Hispanic culture is steeped in conservative Catholicism, a tradition that proscribes the use of condoms and so condemns homosexuality that the Spanish language contains no word for homosexual that is not pejorative.

"In order to be able to communicate about AIDS, you have to talk about topics that are so taboo they aren't even openly discussed among spouses," said Dr. Raphael Tavares, professor of community psychiatry at New York's Columbia Presbyterian Hospital. (Goodman, 1987)[56]

The *New England Journal of Medicine* reported some further disturbing research:

A study of military recruits found that equal numbers of men and women were infected by AIDS in some areas of the United States. . . .

The researchers said the incidence of the disease was highest in densely populated urban areas. . . .

The researcher said that 3.89 of every 1,000 black applicants overall tested positive for the virus compared to 0.88 of every 1,000 whites. (Reuter, 1987)[57]

However one feels about sexual standards, the writing is on the wall. Any ethnic or social group that engages in high risk sex is naturally, scientifically increasing its possibility of encountering the AIDS virus. Premarital and extramarital sex increase exposure risks.

"Latin lovers" and all sexual liberals who have multiple sexual relationships simply increase their chances of contracting AIDS. Unfortunately, those people can pass their contracted AIDS virus on to faithful husbands, wives, lovers, and unborn children.

Although we are discussing particular minorities because they do have a disproportionately high incidence of AIDS, it would serve us well to remember that anyone who engages in unsafe sex is at risk. The Chairman of the Board is no less susceptible to the AIDS virus if he engages in sex with an AIDS carrier than anyone else. Exposure to the AIDS virus through needles, sex, and other risk encounters would greatly increase anyone's chances of getting AIDS.

But blacks and Hispanics present some particular problems at this time. First, and by far most significantly, they are already high risk groups, particularly if they reside in cities. They simply have a higher chance of coming into contact with the AIDS virus. They live in a cultural setting in which the AIDS virus is also living.

Second, as American groups they are generally less educated and informed concerning AIDS. And as lower socio-economic groups they have far fewer resources available to them.

Hispanics and segments of the black community share many of the same problems where AIDS is concerned. Both groups tend to be poor, racially stigmatized and less well-educated, and if they have access to any health care, it is largely inferior. These factors are reflected in AIDS survival rates: Whites live an average of 22 months after diagnosis, non-whites an average of five months. (Boodman, 1987)[56]

When we discuss blacks and Hispanics in numerical and/or abstract terms, it is easy to forget that we are talking about American family members and American families. They can wind up about as far removed in our minds as "voting blocks."

But that is not what we are talking about. We are talking about real, live people who without high incidence of AIDS, were experiencing severe economic problems:

> Minorities bear a disproportionate share of hardship burdens. Blacks, who represented 10 per cent of the total work force in 1979, and 16 per cent of those experiencing unemployment, accounted for 15 per cent of the severe hardship IIE [Inadequate Individual Earnings], 22 per cent of the IFE [Inadequate Family Earnings], and 28 per cent of the IFI [Inadequate Family Income]. The black shares of the severe hardship deficits were 15, 26, and 30 per cent, respectively. While the black shares of the moderate hardship were somewhat lower, the majority of black work force participants had individual earnings below the hardship standard, or 150 per cent of the minimum wage for their hours of availability.
>
> The chances of experiencing unemployment during the year were 165 per cent higher for blacks than whites; and the chances of having individual earnings below the minimum wage equivalent were 151 per cent higher. But only a third of the whites with Inadequate Individual Earnings were in families with Inadequate Family Earnings, compared to almost two-thirds of the blacks in the IIE. (Taggart, 1982)[58]

That employment study showed that Hispanics fared a little better than blacks but significantly worse than whites in U.S. employment. Pre-AIDS-impact, our minorities were experiencing economic problems.

Now with AIDS progressively hitting urban minorities, the remaining American working families will have to cover the economic costs. Those costs to American families will include not only health and welfare costs. The healthy families will also need to make up for the lost productivity among the sick minorities. The increasing load of minorities' dependent children, some of whom will be AIDS victims, also will drain our economic system and return little future productivity.

The Impact Will Be Astounding

As AIDS cases progressively increase, the economic burdens created by AIDS will be like nothing any of us has ever seen. Since all work that produces anything of economic value ultimately comes from our workers, healthy American families and individual family members will have to produce the work that supports AIDS costs.

The better informed that American families are before the AIDS economic onslaught, the more present prevention and future economic preparation they can plan and implement. If we allow the blind to drive our economic vehicle, we are certain to wreck ourselves.

A SPECIAL GROUP: RETIREES

Everyone has been so concerned with sexually active age groups in the United States that another significant group has been virtually ignored - retirees. AIDS, of course, is a predominant concern of sexually active age groups, ages teens through 50's. But it is not because retirees as a group are sexually inactive that they have been mostly ignored concerning AIDS.

Sexually active retirees generally tend to have monogamous sexual relationships. That almost totally eliminates their risks of contracting AIDS - although blood transfusions, etc., still place them at risk. Retirees just tend to engage in safe sexual practices; thus, they have been ignored concerning the vast majority of AIDS related issues.

However, retirees are at risk, serious risk. But it is not the AIDS virus that directly threatens them. Retirees are and will increasingly be threatened by the economic impacts of AIDS.

In President Reagan's fiscal 1989 budget, we find these costs:

Social Security and Medicare

1987: $282.5 Billion
1988: $298.6 Billion
1989: $317.8 Billion
1990: $342.2 Billion

As we will discuss, Social Security, Medicare, and all other forms of retirement benefits and programs are at risk due to AIDS.

Social Security and Medicare

The Social Security Act of 1935 began our national economic approach to financial security for retirees. Employee/employer Social Security costs were comparatively much less then. People did not live as many years as they do now. And we had far more rural dwellers, intact nuclear families, and extended family economic arrangements then.

The social and economic dependency issues differed greatly in the 1930's from the economic dependency issues of the 1980's and 1990's. During the 30's, 40's, and 50's, many Americans ended up not so much retired as job-changed. Because of the far more typical extended family economic arrangements, many retirees continued to contribute work to the overall family economy.

Present and Future Retirees

Rather than using statistical information from a variety of sources, we chose to use a consistent data base from the Life Insurance Marketing and Research Association, Inc. LIMRA is the not-for-profit research trade association of the insurance industry. Therefore, each statistical data base is consistent throughout this discussion.

Anything quoted throughout this section that has a page number beside it is from *The Retirement Markets: Overview and Outlook*, Project Director: Dorothy F. Murray; Editor: Valerie C. Barker, LIMRA, 1986.[59]

Retirees of the 30's–50's could be found babysitting, cleaning and/or repairing family members' houses, gardening, ranching, sewing, etc. Although many of those retirees necessarily reduced the number of hours they worked, they were still contributing work to many family budgets - even if they did not receive a salary for that work.

Since so many retirees continued to work, their work continued to contribute to our overall economy. That directly reduced the demand for economic support from the rest of our economy. Social Security was supplemental, not originally the basis for most retirement support.

But our social and economic environments have substantially changed since then:

TABLE II

Sources of Retirement Income - 1962 and 1984

Per cent of units* aged 65 and over with income from particular source

	1962	1984
Social Security	73%	91%
Income from assets	54	68
Earnings	36	21
Private pensions	9	24
Government employee pensions	5	14

*A unit is a married couple living together or a non-married person. Thus, two non-married or unrelated people living together are counted as two units.

Source: *Income of the Population 55 and Over. 1984.* Social Security Administration

In 1984, 56 per cent of those 65 and older received only one retirement pension - Social Security. The 1984 median income for those who received more than one retirement pension ($15,850) was more than double the income received by those with income only from Social Security ($7,140).

The Social Security Administration also looked at the sources of aggregate income for those 65 and over (Table III). Note the reliance on Social Security benefits across all groups, especially single men and women. While 8 per cent of those 65 and over received some income from assets, income from that source represented just 28 per cent of the aggregate income [p. 30].

TABLE III

Sources of 1984 Aggregate Income for Those Aged 65 and Over

	All units	Married couples	Single men	Single women
Social Security	38%	34%	40%	45%
Earnings	16	21	14	6
Assets	28	27	24	33
Public/private pensions	15	17	18	12
Other	3	1	4	4
	100%	100%	100%	100%

Source: *Income of the Population 55 and Over. 1984.* Social Security Administration

As we can see, Americans who worked and qualified for Social Security retirement benefits are relying more and more on Social Security for their retirement incomes.

As extended families and nuclear families have broken down, retirees have progressively been forced to turn to social and economic support provided by governmental agencies. Although retired individuals' personal families have less and less to do with their retired members' economic support, more and more American families are supporting retired people through individual, family, and business taxes.

When Social Security began, Social Security deductions were comparatively low in proportion to the earned wages from which they were deducted. However, Social Security wage deductions have dramatically increased over the years. Several reasons for the Social Security wage deduction increases exist. However, for our discussion, two contributing factors are of major concern.

Lost Liquidity

After the Crash of 1929 and the Great Depression, the United States had suffered so much economically that its citizens became economically conservative. The Depression generation learned to work, work, work, and save, save, save. They not only worked and produced more but they also saved more of their productivity.

That American economic conservatism continued for some time. Even after World War II, Americans continued an economic tradition of (1) working as a population - social services and welfare costs of all types were much lower than presently; and (2) saving as individuals, family groups, and businesses.

National productivity was often invested in the "American Dream" - family homes - or invested in either new equipment, research and development, new plants, or entirely new American industries. In short, U.S. liquidity was invested in economic growth.

Even through the 1950s the United States had a highly liquid economy. Then came credit, more and more credit. A description of consumer credit from the 1969 *Encyclopedia Americana* indicates the difference between even the attitudes of the 1960s towards credit and our present day attitudes:

> CONSUMER CREDIT . . . is a lending practice by which a consumer obtains goods, services, or cash for immediate use in return for a promise to repay in the future. . . . When a family head borrows cash from a small-loan company or a bank, it is a consumer credit transaction. The charge accounts that a family has are another kind of consumer credit. Credit for a home purchase may be regarded as consumer credit, but its character is so specialized that most authorities treat it separately.
>
> Consumer credit is used for personal consumption. This distinguishes consumer credit from *business credit* [Fischer's italics], which is used for productive purposes.
>
> Consumer credit is largely an American development. . . . Outside the United States consumer credit is far less important.
>
> Total consumer credit outstanding in the United States increased from about $6 billion in 1945 to about $87 billion **20 year later**. (Fischer, 1969)[60]

Today, most all middle and upper income U.S. families have credit cards, or at least have had them. Even cashing a check is difficult in our society if you do not have a credit card. The American economy has become generally a consumer economy. Some "Economic Forecasting Benchmarks for 1988," by Rostvold[28]:

> Savings Out Of Disposable Income 6%
> Net Change in Installment
>   Credit Outstanding .... $50 Billion

Americans are not saving as they once did. They are not even spending as they once did. In our present economy, Americans are borrowing against future earnings to spend today.

That is exactly what happened to our Social Security system. Social Security was established as a prepaid, supplemental retirement program. Proceeds from Social Security payments by wage earners were to fund future retirement benefits that those wage earners would receive. It was supposed to operate much the same as present day private retirement programs have for unions, schools, etc.

But that is not what happened. Over time, proceeds from workers that were supposed to fund their future retirement benefits got spent. As workers contributed to Social Security, their Social Security payments were not invested and saved for their future Social Security benefit payments. Instead, the money was spent making Social Security payments to other people who had retired.

Future Social Security Problems

At least three principal reasons exist for the problems Social Security will face after the turn of the century.

1. Our population is living longer.

2. Inflation outstripped the workers' contributed capital pool.

3. Our government - and probably no one else, either - could not calculate the increasing Social Security payments that were caused by "cost of living" payment increases over the years.

Our Increasingly Older Population

Americans are simply living longer. Better diet and health care have significantly increased the American life span.

> Between 1960 and 1980, the population 65 years and older grew twice as fast as the general U.S. population. This group will increase by 35 per cent between 1980 and 2000.

> Life expectancy for women is now 78.2 years and for men, 70.9 years. Demographers estimate that life expectancy will jump to 81.1 years for women and 73.4 years for men by the year 2000.
>
> In 1935, the birth year of Social Security, the average person who retired at age 65 spent 12 years in retirement. Today, people retire earlier and spend an average of 16 years in retirement [p. 8].

As Americans are living longer, they are also using up their earned/saved productivity. All of their work that produced the savings for retirement have a much greater chance of being spent if they live 75 years rather than 65 years.

We are certainly not "knocking" retired people spending whatever they have saved [One of the authors, Browning, is 70 years old]. However, used up work is just used up. That earned work savings is not available for investment in anything else.

The point is that the United States has spent its liquidity. Individuals, families, businesses, and our government do not have savings to cover unexpected economic catastrophes while trying to meet other obligations that it/they are already committed to meet.

Social Security will hit tremendous, perhaps unsurmountable, problems as AIDS costs increase. What will happen when all the mounting AIDS costs hit our presently deficit budget? We do not believe that even if "Peter tries to rob Paul" it will work: "Paul" is broke, too!

Overall, today's social security system is vastly different from the system established over 50 years ago. Then, the retired population was small compared with the work force, and at $30, so was the maximum annual tax [p. 22].

> In 1950 Social Security paid 28 per cent of all retirement, disability, and survivor benefits in the United States. By 1980 the system's share of the benefit payments more than doubled, while public and private pension plans' shares decreased [p. 21].
>
> As the population ages, there will be fewer workers to support each retiree. The lower worker-to-retiree ratio may affect the Social Security benefits future retirees receive. Therefore, consumers must take steps now to become less dependent on the Social Security system and more dependent on themselves for retirement funds [p. 10].

When we include AIDS demands in this United States picture, the scene is awful. What we will be seeing is not just "fewer workers to support each retiree" but also more and more retirees returning to work to help support the overwhelming national costs of AIDS.

Everything discussed regarding present retirees also applies to future retirees. However, future retirees may very well have all those problems compounded. Future retirees who are presently working may be hit so hard by AIDS costs while they are still working that little or nothing will be left to save for retirement.

Workers of today must support AIDS costs. Past savings to cover escalating AIDS costs certainly do not exist. Therefore, all workers and all American families need to become knowledgeable concerning the economic threats of AIDS now. Otherwise, little hope for retirement for our general population exists. We will all be too busy and economically "strapped" supporting our AIDS victims to plan for and have retirement resources if we wait too long.

LIMRA does an excellent job of summarizing the present retirement situation. Therefore, their following research summary will be used.

Why People Are Not Saving Enough For Retirement

The American Council of Life Insurance commissioned a 1981 study that surveyed 1,000 Americans about the adequacy of their personal financial preparations for retirement. The survey found that while 63 per cent of those surveyed feel they are saving too little, an even higher per cent - 72 per cent - say their savings for retirement are inadequate. Almost half of those surveyed believe they won't be able to afford to retire. Half of the group studied (51 per cent) indicate that no money is being put aside for retirement in their households, while another 21 per cent say that less money is being put aside than is necessary. At the time of the 1981 survey, inflation influenced why people were not setting aside adequate retirement funds.

The survey also found that "the financial pressures on working Americans lead many of them to question whether the main breadwinner in their household will be able to afford retirement. While 50 per cent feel that retirement will be possible, a substantial 44 per cent feel it will not be." [p. 37]

TABLE IV

Why People Are Putting No Money or Not Enough Money Aside for Retirement

Reason	
Other expenses make saving for retirement difficult.	83%
An employer pays for a pension or retirement plan that will help pay for retirement.	29
Current savings are already adequate to cover or help pay for retirement.	10
Social Security will cover all or most retirement needs.	8

*Based on the 51 per cent of working Americans who are not putting money aside for retirement as well as the 21 per cent who are putting less money aside than they feel is necessary.

Source: *American Council of Life Insurance*

The main conclusions of a 1981 survey of 700 full-time workers, conducted for Chemical Bank of New York, are that "The high costs of living, inflation, and a crisis of confidence in Social Security are combining to force workers to rely increasingly on personal savings for their retirement 'nest egg.' However, while most people are in need of greater personal savings for retirement, the majority also say they are falling short in setting aside enough to meet future retirement needs." Here are some highlights of the survey:

• Most employees expect that they will have to dig deep into their personal savings when they retire, and they doubt that Social Security will be there when they need it.

- Employees have the most confidence in their own personal savings, as opposed to Social Security and pension plans.

- Employees find the [then] new individual retirement accounts to be a particularly attractive way of building their retirement nest egg.

Attitudes on Pensions and Retirement

In 1978 Louis Harris conducted a national cross-section survey that focused on American attitudes toward pensions and retirement. Nearly 1,700 current and retired employees of 212 companies were surveyed. There are differences in the ways those surveyed responded, based on whether they were receiving pension benefits.

When asked about their standard of living, "less than adequate" was the response of 56 per cent of those not receiving pension benefits, compared with 23 per cent of those receiving pension benefits.

TABLE V

Adequacy of Standard of Living Among Retirees

	Retirees	Receiving pension benefits	Not receiving pension benefits
More than adequate	12%	16%	8%
Adequate	46	60	35
Less than adequate	42	23	56
Not sure	*	1	--
Number of respondents	396	297	96

Table does not total 100 per cent because of rounding and multiple responses.

*Less than 1/2 of 1 per cent

Source: *1979 Study of American Attitudes Toward Pensions and Retirement*

Fifty-six per cent of all retirees who do not receive pension benefits have "less than adequate" standards of living.

Many retirees feel that their financial plans do not meet their current needs. The Harris survey showed that only 29 per cent of retirees said they had done enough pre-retirement planning. Table VI further breaks down the responses of those who are currently retired. Note the differences between those who are and are not receiving pension benefits [p. 38].

TABLE VI

Amount of Planning for Retirement

	Total	Receiving pension benefits	Not receiving pension benefits
Enough	29%	42%	20%
Some but not enough	26	25	27
Far too little	10	9	10
No planning at all	34	22	42
Not sure	*	1	--
Number of respondents	395	295	95

Table does not total 100 per cent because of rounding and multiple responses.

*Less than 1/2 of 1 per cent

Source: *1979 Study of American Attitudes Toward Pensions and Retirement*

Table VII shows that 56 per cent of the retirees who did little or no retirement planning indicated that their income was less than adequate.

Over half of all retirees who did "little or no retirement planning" have "less than adequate" incomes.

The Harris study also surveyed current workers about the amount of retirement planning they had done. The responses of those aged 35 and over are of special interest. Approximately one fourth had done "no planning at all" and 4 in 10 had done "some but not enough considering present age." [p. 39].

TABLE VII

Retirement Planning and Income Adequacy

	Total	Enough	Retirement planning Some but not enough	Far too little or none
More than adequate	13%	23%	5%	11%
Adequate	46	67	43	33
Less than adequate	41	10	52	56
Not sure	*	--	1	--
Number of respondents	405	116	104	180

Table does not total 100 per cent because of rounding and multiple responses.

*Less than 1/2 of 1 per cent
Source: *1979 Study of Amercian Attitudes Toward Pensions and Retirement*

TABLE VIII

Amount of Planning for Retirement

	Total	18-24	Age 25-34	35-49	50-64
Enough considering present age	33%	21%	30%	34%	38%
Some but not enough considering present age	37	24	36	40	42
No planning at all	30	54	34	26	20
Not sure	*	1	1	*	*
Number of respondents	1,330	150	379	431	339

Table docs not total 100 per cent because of rounding and multiple responses.

*Less than 1/2 of 1 per cent
Source: *1979 Study of Amercian Attitudes Toward Pensions and Retirement*

One fourth of all workers aged 35-49 have done "no [retirement] planning at all; 4 in 10 workers aged 50–64 have done 'some but not enough considering present age.' "

The Harris study also asked participants how much income they thought would be required after retirement. Almost 6 in 10 of those surveyed indicated that they "have not given any thought" to the amount of money required. What may be even more surprising, 48 per cent of those 50 to 64 years of age - the group closest to retirement - responded that they had not given any thought to how much money they would need when they retired.

TABLE IX

Thought Given to Amount of Money Required After Retirement

	Total	18-24	25-34	35-49	50-64
Have given thought	36%	22%	31%	37%	45%
Have not given any thought	58	73	64	56	48
Not sure	6	5	4	7	6
Number of respondents	1,297	148	367	423	335

Table does not total 100 per cent because of rounding and multiple responses.

Source: *1979 Study of Amercian Attitudes Toward Pensions and Retirement*

An effective financial plan must provide for an adequate retirement income. What makes saving for retirement difficult, however, is that financial plans are constantly threatened by competing needs, such as the purchase of and/or upgrading of a home, investment opportunities, and the cost of children's education. Therefore, it takes many years to accumulate funds that will furnish an adequate retirement income. To ensure that these funds do accumulate, consumers must make financial plans on a long-term basis. This lengthy time frame also provides opportunities for

> adjustments in the plan, as competing needs arise and individual goals shift or change [p. 41].
>
> Effective financial retirement planning for many people has not yet been accomplished. The fact that 56 per cent of those 65 and older received income in 1984 from only one retirement pension - Social Security - indicates that there is a long way to go in planning for an adequate income in retirement. While more retirees are receiving income from private pension plans than they have in the past, only 24 per cent of those 65 and over cite private pensions as an income source. Further, the amount of the annual pensions are low. The attitudes of the young professionals cited in Chapter 8 should be of concern: 74 per cent indicated that they "are in fair or poor shape financially for retirement," and 73 per cent "have difficulties saving for retirement [p. 42]."

As we can see from that research, most Americans are not fortunate enough to be working for companies that provide employer-paid retirement programs. Furthermore, most Americans are not saving adequately to provide for their retirement.

In our economic system that has already been stretched to the limits, we have definite indications that social, health, and welfare programs will fail to receive further support. Nationally and in large cities it is worse than nothing available. With all of the deficit spending that has been going on, we are in the red. Economic resources are not and will not be available to support retirees.

AIDS costs will really exacerbate all of our economic woes. Potential retirees, no less than any other group, will be hit too.

Everything discussed regarding present retirees also applies to future retirees. However, future retirees may very well have all those problems compounded. Future retirees who are presently working may be hit so hard by AIDS costs while they are still working that little or nothing will be left to save for retirement.

Workers of today must support AIDS costs. Past savings to cover escalating AIDS costs certainly do not exist. Therefore, all workers and all American families need to become knowledgeable concerning the economic threats of AIDS now. Otherwise, little hope for retirement for our general population exists. We will all be too busy and economically strapped supporting our AIDS victims to plan for and have retirement resources if we wait too long.

Medicare

AIDS issues seem so far removed from present and future retirees' lives that little thought and study have been given to AIDS related retiree issues. However, it could serve us well to expand "the chicken in every pot" economic discussion. When a small family has a chicken in its dinner pot, a lot of protein is available to all the family members. But when you have a family reunion and only one chicken is boiling in the cauldron for the entire extended family, everyone ends up with inadequate nourishment.

That is what is going to happen with present and future retirees. We have one national economic pot. We have one and only one source of "nourishment" to put in that pot - American workers' earnings.

To those who would begin to argue that we have a great influx of foreign capital, we simply reply: No foreign capital would be invested in the United States if we were not one of the most productive countries in the world. Foreign countries do not invest in bankrupt countries. All productivity that makes America economically great falls on American workers and American business.

As AIDS cases and the need for economic support increase, not only Social Security and other governmental forms of retirement support will be threatened but also national and local health care programs will be undermined.

Medicaid and Medicare are already directly involved in AIDS care and costs.

> The government says that 40% of AIDS victims are eventually served by Medicaid and Medicare (the programme for the elderly), though many of them exhaust their savings first. Medicaid will spend some $400m–800m on AIDS care out of $2 billion–3 billion in costs; it expects spending to go up by half next year. Up to now it has covered about 23% of the total medical spending on AIDS, a proportion that varies sharply from area to area. (*The Economist*, 1987)[61]

Another article expands our information and paints an even gloomier picture.

Medicaid Spending on AIDS to Increase Sixfold by 1992, Health Official Says

WASHINGTON-Medicaid spending on AIDS will jump sixfold to $2.4 billion annually by fiscal 1992 from $400 million this year, a top federal health official told members of President Reagan's AIDS Commission at their first public meeting.

Federal funds will have to pay for more than half the expenditures of the Medicaid program serving about 40% of the acquired immune deficiency syndrome population nationwide and 65% of the patients in some high-incidence areas such as New York City. The balance will be paid by the states, as in all Medicaid funding.

"To care for all these cases, we are facing some staggering health care costs over the next several years," said William Roper, administrator for the Health Care Financing Administration, which oversees Medicaid and Medicare programs. "It may surprise you, but the federal government is the major payer for health care for AIDS patients." (Davidson, 1987)[62]

Presently, Medicare benefits look as if they may be improving:

> America's elderly will be protected from the financial ruin of serious illness under a historic expansion of the Medicare program now being negotiated in a House and Senate conference committee.
>
> The Senate voted 86–11 to pass the catastrophic health legislation Tuesday evening. The House version passed 302–127 on July 23.
>
> Medicare now pays full hospital bills for only 60 days a year, after a one-day deductible of $544. The catastrophic health expansion provides 365 day-a-year coverage after a one-day deductible.
>
> In another change, the new program will cap out-of-pocket doctor bills at somewhere between $1,043 and $1,850 a year. Medicare now pays only 80 per cent of doctor bills, no matter how high they rise. The legislation also provides for a Medicare benefit for outpatient prescription drugs. (*The Albuquerque Tribune*, October 28, 1987)[63]

Although differences remain between the two measures, it's now all but certain that Congress soon will enact legislation limiting patient outlays for Medicare-covered hospital and physician services. And, for the first time, it will put a ceiling on out-of-pocket costs for outpatient prescription drugs and safeguard against "spousal impoverishment" - changes that represent substantial broadening of Medicare. (Coleman, 1988)[64]

But before we are lulled into a false sense of security, we need to examine some other important Medicare information:

In Poor Health
Small Rural Hospitals
Struggle for Survival
Under Medicare Setup

The nation is "wringing excess capacity out of the system," says William Roper, the head of the U.S. Health Care Financing Administration, which administers Medicare, the federal health-insurance program for the elderly. "Medicare isn't able to assure the survival of every hospital," Dr. Roper says. "Our objective ought to be to have an efficient health-care system."

. . . But that summer, a Congress concerned with spiraling health costs passed the Medicare Reform Act, the legislation that required the flat-rate system.

"If a person dies in 13 hours, you get paid the same as if they'd stayed 13 weeks," says Garland Hall, a family-practice physician here. "Death has become the most cost-effective treatment." (Bean, 1988)[65]

Medical care cost problems well pre-date AIDS. But AIDS will make those problems far worse. Questions presently being asked will increase, and the need for answers will accelerate.

Medicare does not begin to answer all the medical care cost problems for retirees, nor anyone else.

While catastrophic health care legislation is still languishing in Congress, growing attention already is being focused on the next issue: Long-term care of the disabled outside of hospitals.

Even though such care is the biggest health-related financial burden most elderly people will face, many don't realize that Medicare pays for less than 2% of nursing-home expenses and private insurance picks up only about 1%. That leaves a lot of elderly people in a financial bind, since the average annual cost of a nursing home stay is $22,000. (Goodman, 1987)[66]

Freedberg points out that "1.5 million Americans live in nursing homes." He further uses the American Health Care Association's estimates and tells us about the occupancy of nursing homes: 93% White; 6% Black; and 1% Other. (Freedberg, 1988)[67]

Those numbers are very informative. They indicate what is American reality: Middle class - wealthy Americans end up in nursing homes. They can afford the costs. However, our lower socio-economic groups, particularly our minorities, cannot afford such care.

The same groups in which AIDS case loads are increasing are the same socio-economic groups that cannot afford nursing home and/or health care. As AIDS spreads in those at-risk lower socio-economic groups, all other tax supported social, health, and welfare programs will be vying for the same support out of our single economic American pot.

"Case Management" will increasingly become a reality for persons not directly paying their own medical bills. Due to specific insurances cases that cost exorbitant amounts, some insurance companies have begun case management. That usually leads to more reasonable and more payable medical bills. But if not well managed, case management can lead to poorer care. (Ricklefs, 1987)[68]

Governmental case management is likely to become increasingly disease specific as well as case specific. With the progression of AIDS, governmental health care agencies will have little choice. Present and future retirees need to be aware of their own position as decisions regarding national health care are made. As always, the silent will be ignored.

IMPACT OF AIDS ON BUSINESS AND WORKERS

All businesses have already begun to be affected by AIDS. Even if a company is unaware of the AIDS impact, the growing magnitude of the AIDS public costs have hit all businesses to some degree.

As AIDS public costs mount, taxes will continue to increase for business and workers alike. The costs of AIDS in human life and economic wealth will increasingly come to be directly experienced by everyone.

Companies now, however, are being affected. And it does not matter whether we examine for-profit or non-profit businesses. They are all being affected. As for-profit companies pay more taxes, that reduces their cash flow that was available for donations and non-profit organizations' membership dues.

Between the Tax Reform Act of 1986 and the cost of AIDS, non-profit and charitable organizations will also have decreasing revenues. The "business meetings" that churches and other charitable and non-profit organizations have are for just that--business. The monies they receive are no less part of our economy than for-profit monies. Therefore, for our economic discussion, any organization that has income is threatened as a business.

Just as for-profit businesses, charitable and service organizations with income will have their cash flow affected. AIDS will, because of the growing cases and increasing AIDS costs, progressively decrease all businesses' income.

Even Fritz Perls was economically wise enough to note, "A balanced budget is one in which credit and debit add up to zero, whether the budget deals with pennies or millions." (Perls, 1976)[67] Any and all businesses cognizant of present and increasing AIDS costs can prepare more wisely and at least have some hope of a balanced budget.

"Companies say housing and AIDS will also join the list of top five social concerns over the next five years." (*The Wall Street Journal*, December 3, 1987.)[68] We believe that AIDS will be THE concern in the next five years. As cash flow increasingly becomes the major concern for all types of business, business focus will be on AIDS.

The same economic costs of AIDS that will hit businesses will also hit the workers' pocket books and bank accounts. Fritz was right. It does not matter whether we deal in hundreds, thousands, millions, or billions. Credit and debit have to add up to zero for a worker's, business's, or nation's budget to balance.

Initially, the two major concerns for business will be focused on the public fear of AIDS and increasing insurance costs. From developing AIDS related problems in the work place, AIDS policy issues will arise. Productivity will continually decline, and AIDS disability cases will increase. As AIDS continues to become a clearly heterosexual disease, all aspects of business will be involved.

A few, very few, businesses will increase their economic profits directly due to AIDS. The vast majority of businesses will suffer increasing costs because of AIDS. Even the businesses that avoid many of the AIDS costs, because they have made early, wise policy decisions, cannot avoid the increasing taxation. All governmental levels will necessarily increase taxes over time.

Through time, workers will increasingly be asked to increase both their efficiency and productivity. The request for increased efficiency and productivity will not be caused by greed, however. The whip that will end up driving us all to work more efficiently, productively, and longer hours will be the whip of necessity.

The AIDS virus will kill and disease so many people that we will have no choice in a few years. But if we make some wise decisions now, we can perhaps avoid some of the economic tragedy to come. It is time for all of business - workers, managers, and owners - to get involved with decisions regarding our AIDS problems.

Public Fear of AIDS

Just about everyone has read articles about AIDS victims houses being burned, rocks being thrown at AIDS victims, swimming pools being drained because someone with AIDS had swum in them, and certainly the social prejudice that AIDS victims face. Compared to what we will be seeing in the future, all of that is a minor beginning.

> "Though international leadership by the World Health Organization has been met with an unusually high degree of multinational cooperation, AIDS has also stimulated a degree of xenophobia and racial friction that, if allowed to grow, could handicap global AIDS control and prevention efforts." (Sabatier, 1987)[69]

Fear of foreigners, things foreign, and racial friction are not limited by national boundaries.

In the United States, fear of culturally "foreign" people and ideas is often seen. Many further claim that our racial friction is merely below the surface, that racial prejudice within our country still exists.

Since homosexuals are in a sense "foreign" to many Americans, fear is often generated by homosexuals' sexual and lifestyle preferences. Combine that with the high incidence of homosexuals' AIDS cases, and you have a precursor of trouble.

The same can be said of racial minorities. Take the pre-existing racial prejudice and combine that with some minorities' high incidence of AIDS and problems can arise.

The AIDS virus itself is psychologically foreign to people. We cannot see it, hear it, touch it or know that we have touched it, smelled it, nor tasted it. It's just out there. And, generally, humans are much better psychologically prepared to deal with something that they can sense in some manner. Sensing the enemy in some manner seems - and usually does - to give us the chance to protect ourselves.

Although many things are available to us to help protect us from AIDS - mainly rigorous sexual discretion - most people aware of the AIDS problem feel in danger. That fear can be invaluable if it leads to protective measures. That fear can also be disruptive if it is partially or mostly based on ignorance.

Ignorance regarding AIDS in the work place can rapidly lead to enormous problems. Fear + Ignorance can cause workers, managers, and business owners a great deal of trouble. Everything from social overreaction against AIDS victims to lost jobs and business bankruptcies can and will occur if all sectors of business do not inform themselves.

The potential problem we see is this: "As [AIDS] infection spreads, the polarization within society between those who are carriers of the virus and those who are not will increase." (Sabatier, 1987)[69]

> Society at large is confronted with psychosocial disruption and its concomitant symbols, causing frank questions and discussions in families, classrooms, civic groups, and churches and presenting a challenge to the limits of what our cultures and subcultures are willing to permit in the struggle to contain AIDS. The issues raised by the effort to control and prevent AIDS go far beyond the communication of information to improve knowledge. AIDS takes the measure of our sexual balance, our prejudices and our integrity, how we love and how we deal with death and dying. (Meyer, 1987)[70]

We are not discussing a future problem. AIDS is THE present problem in the United States:

> Intolerance and abuse of AIDS victims is likely to persist if the uninfected population has any cause to suspect that its safety isn't being protected. Such a backlash is also likely to erupt if the general population comes to believe that it isn't being told the truth, because the facts would put the livelihoods and liberties of AIDS carriers in jeopardy. Civil rights will indeed be threatened if civil-rights politics overwhelms public-health. (*The Wall Street Journal*, September 9, 1987)[71]

> WASHINGTON - Lawyers and health workers urged Congress on Tuesday to pay more attention to the public's rights of protection from AIDS rather than focusing on the civil rights of AIDS victims and carriers. (Associated Press, 1987)[72]

All, not some, of the AIDS problems are present in business situations simply because AIDS victims are in business places. Fear and prejudice are not the least of our AIDS related, AIDS caused problems.

> A clash between the rights of employees suffering from AIDS and those of noninfected co-workers could pose a growing problem for employers, according to a survey of attitudes toward people who have the disease.
>
> The survey, by the Center for Work Performance Problems at the Georgia Institute of Technology, focused on workplaces in its questions. . . .
>
> Two-thirds of the respondents said they would be concerned about using the same bathroom as an AIDS sufferer on the job, 40 per cent were concerned about using the same cafeteria, and 37 per cent said they would not be willing to use the same equipment as an AIDS sufferer. (Smothers, 1988)[73]

Our reason tells us that all AIDS problems will impact all sectors of business. Everyone will be affected by AIDS, not just AIDS victims. But unlike the Black Plague, something can be done about the devastation of AIDS.

Employees and employers can inform themselves concerning AIDS and take appropriate protective actions. The rampant fear in the work place can be mainly dispelled through informed people exchanging information with the uninformed.

Although the work place has never been considered an appropriate place to teach sex education, it certainly is now. AIDS for the general population is almost totally a sexually transmitted disease. As a disease that threatens all of our lives and does not discriminate between work place or non-work place, all aspects of AIDS education need to be discussed in the work place.

Furthermore, an accurate, comprehensive discussion of AIDS transmission can eliminate many of the fears in the work place. Particularly accurate, rational, comprehensive knowledge concerning the risk of contracting AIDS through casual contact can dispel many employers' and employees' fears.

Dr. Walters, of the Canadian Public Health Association, provides one of the best discussions for the general population that we have seen concerning public fear and "perceived risk." (Walters, 1987)[74]

WORK PLACE AIDS:
"The Non-Epidemic"

At the recent Ottawa workshop on **AIDS and the Work Place,** co-sponsored by Health and Welfare Canada and CPHA, a Union leader stated that the constant barrage of terms like "epidemic" and "virus" continues to fuel the public fear the HIV infection can spread in a "flu-like" wave wherever people work, learn or live together.

Medical and nursing leaders also related that it has taken continuing concerted education even in the most experienced city hospitals to quell the fears of staff, patients and families about the risk of infection.

Likewise, educators and business managers tell of disruptions, grievances and pressures to institute ill-founded screening programs and to isolate infected individuals so that the "perceived risk" to others is eliminated.

What are the real risks and problems of HIV infection in the work place? Perhaps the most intense exposure to HIV for workers has occurred in hospitals like the San Francisco General where medical, nursing and lab staff have worked constantly with AIDS patients for over 5 years and unknowingly with infected people and blood for several years before that. Yet, specific studies of the staff have not shown a single HIV infection attributable to these occupational exposures. In fact, worldwide, there have only been about twelve individual cases of health care workers becoming infected by accidental needlesticks and splashes of infected blood on damaged skin.

Such rare occurrences with major exposures indicate that the vast majority of work situations other than hospitals pose no risk of transmission. It cannot be argued that our experience is too short to be sure about this because there have now been numerous surveillance studies in different countries all confirming the work place non-epidemic. This risk can be managed adequately with the introduction of "universal precautions" in the health care setting which requires the precaution of latex gloves as a first step whenever exposure to blood or body fluids is possible.

It is critical that American business recognize the true risk factors. AIDS is NOT generally transmitted through casual contact. The experience in San Francisco General and other places around the world that have been involved with long term AIDS care have taught us that.

But all business needs to know those facts. Employee assistance programs, unions, employers and employees need to know the facts about risk of exposure. Otherwise, fear of AIDS can initially cause more economic disruptions in our society than AIDS itself.

AIDS does and will continue to affect all aspects of business. However, we have some real, concrete choices about dispelling the myths. We can reduce the unfounded, irrational fears by teaching the facts. Moreover, we can reduce even the remote possibilities of AIDS transmission through casual contact by heeding the facts.

The more we know and act on that knowledge, the safer all of us will be.

INSURANCE COSTS

The second area of American business that will experience the most initial impact of AIDS is insurance costs. AIDS will also continue to cause insurance costs to rise for some time to come. The more AIDS victims - the more dying and deaths - the higher insurance rates will go.

Insurance companies are no different than other businesses: Credit and debit must add up to at least zero to have a balanced budget. Since insurance companies are for-profit businesses, they - just as all other for-profit businesses - work and plan to make a profit. Insurance companies' financial well being is founded on a positive cash flow.

However, when an individual's or business's insurance rates significantly rise, the individual worker or business tends to forget the insurance company's for-profit position. Since no way exists for most of us to know personally an insurance company, it is easy for that personally unknown entity to become a scapegoat.

Initially, many employees and employers who have to pay higher insurance premiums will blame the insurance industry. But it is not the insurance industry that is to blame.

Insurance companies are merely passing increasing costs on to the ultimate consumers: You and me. Blaming insurance companies for increased insurance costs is exactly like blaming your local gas station for higher oil prices and gasoline prices. The insurance industry can no more control the growing number of AIDS cases than your local gas station can control escalating oil prices.

The only thing that the insurance industry can do is attempt to control the costs of their AIDS case loads. That is why we see John Hancock run a three-quarter page ad in *The Wall Street Journal*.

Someday soon, every corporation in America will face an AIDS problem.

Your company may or may not have documented AIDS cases right now. But it doesn't really matter, because you undoubtedly will in the future.

AIDS will impact all of us. The problem is here to stay.

So for insurance company and corporation alike, the game has changed and the stakes are almost beyond measure.

Over the next decade, the projected costs of AIDS care for both employers and insurers is staggering. Just in the next five years, the bill could reach $40 billion.

And the projected human costs are even greater because they are incalculable.

Naturally, we don't have all the answers. No one does.

But we are responding. With compassion. With understanding. With intelligence.

How?

We've developed a better way to handle AIDS cases with the help of John Hancock's AIDS Case Management Service.

Specifically this service comprises a national network of registered nurses who coordinate the medical care of employees or dependents with AIDS.

> Working with Hancock consultants and employee benefits personnel, the program effectively reduces costs by seeking alternative forms of care.
>
> Including out-patient clinics. Home health care agencies. Hospice care.
>
> These alternatives can achieve significant savings over the cost of in-hospital stays. They are a smart management option.
>
> But there's an even more important idea here.
>
> Because our AIDS Case Management Service offers much more than cost containment.
>
> By encouraging non-institutional care, it offers AIDS patients more of the one thing they have left to hold onto.
>
> Their dignity.
>
> And there's no way to put a price on that.
> (John Hancock, 1988)[75]

We certainly are not endorsing John Hancock, nor any other insurance company, for that matter. But we all need to be aware of insurance companies' situations concerning the impact of AIDS. No insurance company runs a costly three-quarter page ad for the "hey" of it.

Because AIDS sufferers will increasingly lack personal funds to pay for their care costs, those AIDS costs will be covered by insurance and/or taxes. One way or another, we all will end up sharing in the costs of AIDS care. We will all pay higher insurance premiums, if we have present health insurance and/or death policies with variable rates or new insurance policies. We will all pay higher taxes in the future - our tax hike being directly caused by increasing AIDS costs.

It is just unreasonable to choose the insurance industry as the "fall guy." But worse than that, such reasoning only serves to defocus our vision. Employees and employers alike need to understand the consequences of AIDS on their income sources. AIDS costs will reduce our take home pay and our business profits.

The problems of AIDS case costs is not just the insurance industry's problem; it is all of our problem. And those costs are high and will become astronomical.

Aggressive Marketers Will Pay Price In AIDS Claims: Study

AIDS related deaths from existing policies could cost American life insurers up to $50 billion by the year 2000, according to a new study released by the Society of Actuaries. The study was authored by Michael J. Cowell and Walter H. Hoskins, actuaries for Worcester, Mass. - based State Mutual Life Ins. Co. of America.

AIDS-Related Deaths Could Surpass 20% Of Future Claims

AIDS Death Claim Tab Could Cost Insurers $50 Billion

(Headlines From *National Underwriter*, August 17, 1987)

Insurance Industry Fears AIDS Threat

WASHINGTON - AIDS poses a serious threat to the insurance industry, and companies must take steps to make sure they can deliver on their benefit commitments even in the face of "worst-case scenario," an industry group said Monday.

The risk of mortality for carriers of the AIDS virus is so high that "they cannot be considered insurable for life insurance," the American Academy of Actuaries said in a report.

A 35-year-old male with AIDS has about the same life expectancy as a non-infected 70-year-old man, said the report by the academy's committee on life insurance.

"Put another way," it said, "for each $1,000 of life insurance issued unknowingly to an HIV carrier, the insurance company is assuming roughly a $515 unfunded and unanticipated liability."

The federal Center for Disease Control estimates that AIDS will strike 270,000 people and kill 179,000 by the end of 1991. (*Albuquerque Journal*, September 29, 1987)[77]

ACLI Study Sets 1986 AIDS Claims At $290M
(Ness, 1987)[78]

AIDS Is Growing Problem For Group Insurers

A North American Re survey of group life and health insurers disclosed that the average AIDS group life insurance death claim is about $38,000, or 2.7 times the average non-AIDS claim, which is about $14,000.

The 80 group insurers which participated in the survey had a total of more than 11,000 AIDS claims for group life, medical, disability, and credit business in the 2.5 years between the beginning of 1985 and mid-1987. Group AIDS claims increased by 60 per cent from 1985 to 1986 and by 47 per cent from 1986 to 1987 on an annualized basis, the survey reported.

More than 40 per cent of the surveyed companies reported they are doing some form of testing for AIDS in group coverages that are individually underwritten. (*National Underwriter*, December 21, 1987)[79]

When we consider the present AIDS claim at "2.7 times the average non-AIDS claim," we can begin to understand the present situation of the insurance industry. Then when we further know that the insurance industry found $290 million in 1986 AIDS claims and projects "$50 billion by the year 2000," we can see what they are facing. Furthermore, we can trust the accuracy of those present and projected numbers. Those numbers came from the insurance industry and were presented for the insurance industry, not the general reading public.

Most Insurance Firms Screen for AIDS

WASHINGTON-Screening of health insurance applicants to detect AIDS virus is a common practice among insurance companies and health maintenance organizations, according to a congressional study released Wednesday.

The Congressional Office of Technology Assessment said its survey of commercial insurers, Blue Cross and Blue Shield plans and HMOs found that most insurers ask AIDS-related questions on applications and require health histories from an applicant's physician.

The report said 51, or 86 per cent, of the 62 commercial insurers who responded to the survey either screen or plan to screen individual applicants for the HIV infection. Forty-one already do and another 10 plan to start the tests. Eleven of 15 Blue Cross plans surveyed either screen or plan to screen, as do eight of 16 responding HMOs. (*Albuquerque Journal*, February 18, 1988)[80]

The insurance industries' developing policies and positions certainly are not a conspiracy against AIDS victims. Insurance companies are just wisely attempting to survive, and survive with a profit as all other for-profit businesses would do.

Everything that is AIDS related and hitting the insurance companies will profoundly affect American business. United States employees and employers will pick up the AIDS costs. As AIDS costs escalate in all areas, it will be all of us paying the tab.

Bankrupt businesses do not send out bills after they are gone. They are simply done and gone. Insurance companies are a vital part of our economy. Frankly, we are glad that they have the sense and foresight to attempt to protect their economic security - we sure would not want an insurance policy with any company that did not try to protect their economic solvency. Insurance companies contribute to our overall economy in many ways.

AIDS effect on insurance companies is and will continue to be obvious. However, some of the ripple effects of AIDS on other sectors of the economy may not be so immediately apparent. A tidal wave of unanticipated insurance claims could destroy some insurance companies. Insurance claims are not paid by bankrupt companies. Therefore, the entire insurance industry has and will continue to prepare for the AIDS crises.

But insurance companies do more than just insure people's health and lives. As a group, insurance companies manage more retirement plan portfolios than any other single business group. Insurance companies probably have some of the most astute managers and the most investment information for long term, less speculative and therefore more secure investments.

As the older members of our working population are forced to "take up the slack" in production, our older members will also be faced with dwindling retirement security. Many people will need secure retirement programs. Social Security is already threatened. Social Security is already borrowing against the future retirement benefits of workers to pay retired workers.

The over-50 workers will be faced with sharing the costs for supporting our dying population and their children. And while the over-50 workers are sharing the brunt of social welfare costs, they will have their own economic security further undermined. Many of those who can put something aside for retirement will need reliable, secure retirement programs in which to invest.

After working all day, most workers just do not have time to run some type of complicated, sophisticated investment program for their retirement. Insurance companies can serve us well by running secure, sophisticated retirement investment programs.

We can start listening to insurance companies. Because of their profit motive and enlightened self interest, insurance companies are tracking AIDS developments and the economic impacts of AIDS like no one else. Of course, insurance companies are studying AIDS because it is hitting and will continue to hit their industry so hard. But AIDS will eventually have just as great an impact on all of us.

We have two existing protections from insurance company manipulation of the American public:

1. Competition - just plain old American free enterprise. Each insurance company competes against other insurance companies for a market share. The consumer - everyday working Americans - selects from whom to buy from among the competitors. Any insurance company that tried to take advantage of American insurance buyers would rapidly get caught by both the insurance buyer - individuals, businesses, and government agencies - and competing insurance companies. You can be sure that competing insurance companies would let us all know if some insurance company was trying to "rip us off."

2. Sophisticated Analysts - university economics professors, Wall Street money managers and investors, union economics analysts, city, state, and federal government money managers, heads of corporations, MBAs, and informed citizens. Couple that with

the free press and our guaranteed right to speak. With the available analyses and the American press's willingness (most of the press believes "obligation") to let Americans know what is happening, the United States insurance industry's AIDS information can be trusted.

We are a little too experienced to trust serendipitously any for-profit company or industry. But insurance companies simply are not in the position to manipulate AIDS information and/or insurance rates. Our economic system has too many inherent controls against such actions. We have, therefore, relied on a lot of insurance information. We have also found the insurance industry to be the most consistent, reliable, and comprehensive source of information regarding AIDS.

Insurance companies can help all American business, if we will listen.

Lost Productivity

This will be a short but very sour discussion. The consequences of AIDS-caused lost productivity are incredible, but true. AIDS will cause economic chaos shortly.

Some agreement over time concerning the costs of AIDS-caused lost productivity exists:

> The economic and social consequences of AIDS are only now beginning to be understood. Data from surveys in New York City, Philadelphia and San Francisco suggest that the first 10,000 patients with AIDS reported in the United States will require an estimated 1.6 million days in hospital, resulting in over $1.4 billion in expenditures. An additional $4.8 billion in losses will be incurred for the 8,387 years of lost work from the disability and premature death of these patients.[2] (Meyer, 1987)[81]

> The disease [AIDS] would cost the U.S. $1.25 billion in medical expenses and $4.38 billion in "lost productivity," according to the Center for Disease Control. The estimates were reported Sept. 16 [1985]. (*Facts on File*, November 15, 1985)[82]

Some elementary math provides us with a cost analysis of lost productivity due to AIDS:

TABLE X: LOST PRODUCTIVITY

Meyer's: $1.4 billion in expenditures
          x 3.4
          $4.76 billion

(Meyer's lost work = $4.8 billion)

Facts on File $1.25
                 x 3.5
                 $4.375 billion

(*Fact's* $4.38 billion in "Lost Productivity")

Roughly, that means for every $1 spent on AIDS expenses, $3.4 to $3.5 is lost in work productivity. We ask our readers to choose whatever cost number they think most reliable and multiply that number by $3.4 or $3.5. You will then have a means for determining present and probably near future AIDS-caused lost productivity.

> We are headed where Uganda is ending up:

> A total of 1,138 cases of AIDS have been reported in Uganda, Okware says, about 85% of which occur among the sexually most active age group-men and women in equal numbers between 15 and 40 years of age. These include some of Uganda's most productive adults, in professional and economic terms, and Okware predicts that the impact of AIDS-related deaths among this group could be devastating to the country's welfare. (*Research News*, 1987)[83]

As if all that news were not bad enough, the entire problem of lost productivity is compounded by other factors:

> . . . the contagiousness of those positive for the virus is rising. Over time, the viral load increases in the body of a person carrying HIV, particularly as the immune system begins to falter. The person with this virus gradually becomes more infectious. Those heterosexually exposed over the past few years to people positive for the virus may have encountered a low level of infectiousness compared with those who will have contact with people carrying the virus during the next few years. (Robinson, 1987)[84]

Those findings that "the contagiousness of those positive for the virus is rising" come from the National Institutes of Health study of Finnish men. The findings can only mean that we are becoming progressively more at risk.

But it gets worse:

> Scientists have known for some time that the human immunodeficiency virus (HIV) that causes AIDS enters the central nervous system and remains there. The great majority of AIDS patients experience some mental impairment, and AIDS dementia has recently been included by the Center for Disease Control as a manifestation of the illness.
>
> But researchers were surprised to find that even apparently healthy individuals show definite signs of problems that could harm their judgment severely. (*The Washington Post*, 1987)[85]

If "apparently healthy individuals" who are AIDS carriers have "their judgment severely" affected, our productivity certainly will be influenced. It looks like AIDS can damage productivity in ways never remotely measured.

Long before employers start paying disability costs and taxpayers begin welfare supports to an AIDS victim, our society will start paying for AIDS costs. Indeed, we have already begun paying. The proportional loss of our most productive age group will be carried by employees and employers alike. Our business economy will have to carry the load.

BUSINESS AND OCCUPATIONS AFFECTED BY AIDS

We reviewed numerous industries and the entire *Dictionary of Occupational Titles* (U.S. Labor Department, 1986).[86] Our news is not happy. We could find only very few industries and, therefore, occupations that would not be badly impacted by AIDS.

Some of the most severely affected will, of course, be insurance, medical care of all types, the fashion industry - including advertising by major companies to gay audiences (Alsop, 1988)[87], sexually explicit anything, and through time occupations that are tax supported.

Some exotic, newly developing industries may do well:

A biophysicist at Los Alamos National Laboratory has figured out a way to use laser beams as if they were microscopic tongs to pick up individual live cells less than one-thousandth of an inch thick.

Tudor Buican is now trying to automate the cell manipulation technique, which is expected to be a boon to biologists, immunologists and others in biomedicine.

"Most cell-sorting techniques can only separate out groups of cells, rather than individual cells," Buican said. "The methods that handle individual cells either don't position them very accurately or involve relatively bulky mechanical devices."

Buican's method uses laser light to trap a cell within a beam. The cell will go wherever the beam is pointed. When the laser's intensity is reduced, the cell will drop off. By using two laser beams, Buican can trap the cell at the intersection of the beams, permitting him to move the cell in any direction.

The lasers permit the cell sorting to be done in a completely enclosed container as small as a fingernail. "This eliminates the threat of contamination and is ideal for experiments in space," Buican said. (*Albuquerque Journal*, 1988)[88]

Anything that "eliminates the threat of contamination" will progressively become recognized in AIDS research and treatment. The usefulness and often necessity of preventing AIDS viral contamination will foster the economic growth of specific, unusual industries.

All products and manufacturing of disposable gloves, not merely surgical gloves, will continue to experience growth. "Demand is soaring for surgical, examination and other disposable medical gloves. . . ." (Berkman, 1987)[89]

Not only industries involved with products for and manufacturing of medical gloves will increase their trade, but also businesses associated with cleaning gloves will experience growth. The more aware persons become of the need to protect themselves around body fluids in general, the more cleaning gloves will be sold for health protection. In the near future, we will see cleaning personnel putting on gloves much as medical people do now.

"Companies must educate employees about AIDS to prevent 'groundless hysteria' when a co-worker contracts the deadly disease, the U.S. surgeon general [Koop] said Tuesday." (Associated Press, 1987)[90] Not only companies but schools also must educate their students. As an industry, education should do well; educational demands will increase. However, no one knows exactly what will happen to the birth rate due to AIDS.

Companies such as Clorox that manufacture and distribute household *and* industrial bleach are likely to do well. The reason for that is simple: Ordinary bleach in a 10 part water/1 part bleach solution kills the AIDS virus.

Any industry involved with food - meat packing to restaurants - can use that 10/1 solution to protect against the spread of the AIDS virus.

Although it is highly improbable that the AIDS virus is spread through contact with food at any stage of food preparation, the possibility exists. Furthermore, cleaning with a 10/1 bleach solution is a win-win deal - that bleach solution also kills salmonella bacteria, which cause food poisoning and are pathogenic for man.

Janitorial cleaning solutions containing bleach will also be increasingly used. In any physical area in which body fluids are persistently present - bathrooms, motels and hotels, hospitals, etc. - bleach solutions will increasingly come to be used as disinfectants. (That bleach solution will also kill staph, so we have another win-win deal.)

Companies that manufacture crematory equipment will also probably do well. At first, we thought the entire mortuary business would do well. However, after a lot more analysis, we changed our minds. We are certain that the mortuary industry will experience increased business. But so many problems are associated with AIDS victims' bodies and their burial that we are not sure what is going to happen to the overall burial business.

First, and initially probably the most obvious consideration, AIDS victims' burials will increasingly be paid for by the government. So many AIDS victims will be destitute that taxpayers will have to cover burial costs. Governmental agencies will decide how AIDS victims' bodies are treated. Since burial costs normally exceed cremation costs, more and more AIDS victims will be cremated.

Another factor exists that will compound the incidence of cremation. The AIDS virus is killed at 56 degrees Celsius (132.8 degrees Fahrenheit). Although the thought is morbid [We will be increasingly faced with addressing morbid topics with AIDS.], it is obvious that cremation kills the AIDS virus.

Cremation may significantly decrease the necessity of additional human contact with AIDS victims' bodies. As well, cremation may reduce the overwhelming AIDS costs in at least one tax-supported area.

COMPANY AIDS POLICIES

Rather than bore some of our readers with all of the policy details, we decided to provide our Appendices and a series of title quotes. Appendix A is "Designing a Corporate AIDS Policy" by Corporate Security and Investigations, Inc. Appendix B is "Guidelines for Handling Issues Related to AIDS" by Chevron. Appendix C is "Policy on Assisting Employees with Life-Threatening Illnesses by The Bank of America. (Again, we thank those companies for generously sharing their experience and knowledge with us.)

The headlines and titles of various articles tells much of the AIDS policy story. We have included not only the author's name but also the publication source because that further informs us of the magnitude of the AIDS policy problem.

"Firms Slow to Set Policies On Employees With AIDS"; "Education of Work Force Called Key"; "Area Firms Struggle With AIDS Issue"; "Some Settle Quietly With Fired Patients"; "Some Large Local Firms Begin AIDS Education" (Spolar, *The Washington Post*, September 7, 1987)[91]

"AIDS in the Workplace: What Can Be Done?" (Masi, *Personnel*, July 1987)[92]

"AIDS: Tackling a Tough Problem Policy; Developing a workplace Policy on AIDS may be a complex task." (Meyers & Meyers, *Personnel Administrator*, April 1987)[93]

"Employee Assistance; AIDS Information Clearinghouse Launched by Personnel Journal"; (Magnus, *Personnel Journal*, September 1987)[94]

"AIDS in the Workplace: Public Personnel Management and the Law"; (Elliott & Wilson, *Public Personnel Management*, Fall 1987)[95]

"The Work Environment; A Practical Guide for Dealing with AIDS at Work"; (Waldo, *Personnel Journal*, August 1987)[96]

"When a Worker Gets AIDS; Education is the key to preventing employee panic and fear." (Puckett, *Psychology Today*, January 1988)[97]

"AIDS in the Workplace: Fighting Fear with Facts and Policy"; (Lutgen, *Personnel*, November 1987)[98]

"The Workplace & AIDS: A Guide to Services and Information"; (Magnus, Editor, *Personnel Journal*, October 1987)[99]

"Dealing with AIDS; Above all, the victim needs compassion - and understanding." (Verespej, *Industry Week*, February 1, 1987)[100]

[If anyone wishes to obtain additional AIDS policy information, we recommend any and all of those articles.]

AIDS has created so many serious policy issues that it is amazing. Usually, employers develop policy guidelines. They often include employees in their policy decision making process, but it is most often the employer side that begins the process of policy consideration.

With AIDS policy considerations, that is not always the case. We had several employers tell us that their employees were pushing for some AIDS policy establishment. Particularly with the interviewed employers who had an AIDS case(s) among their employees, fellow employees were often demanding some AIDS policy, and fast.

Many policy questions do not have any answers yet. For example, what can legally be done about seemingly healthy employees who have AIDS or ARC but who may also be suffering mental decline? How and when can and does an employer measure the mental acuity of an employee? How does an employer establish pre-AIDS mental ability and with-AIDS mental ability? What about retarded persons' rights? Are employers who measure mental functions without pre-established baselines discriminating?

"Questions of law, ethics, economics, morality, and social cohesion exacerbate tensions over fatal disease that cannot yet be cured." (Ember, 1987)[101] As you will see through reading in the Appendixes, AIDS questions far outweigh AIDS policy answers.

> Asking the questions, even the right questions, does not seem to solve a lot of the policy issues either. In January 1988, "representatives of some of the country's largest corporations" gathered in Washington and presented "federal officials with their recommendations on how businesses can best prepare for and react to incidents of acquired immune deficiency syndrome in the workplace."
>
> "The report . . . 'AIDS: Corporate America Responds' - is the product of a national conference sponsored last fall by Allstate Insurance Co. . . ."

> The report reminds employers that "all federal and state courts and state agencies have held that AIDS is a handicap entitled to protection [against] discrimination. . . ."

The report cites the Supreme Court's 1987 decision in the case of The School Board of Nassau County vs. Arline. Although that case addressed tuberculosis and not AIDS, the Court's decision extended protection of federal handicap statutes to contagious diseases. Moreover, the report says that testing for antibodies to HIV, the AIDS virus, "is likely to be considered illegal since testing positive for HIV cannot be shown to be related to performance on the job."

Raising a Red Flag

> The legal chapter [of AIDS: Corporate America Responds] raises one red flag that is bound to spark arguments. It cautions that companies that hand out written AIDS policies to all employees may create a new class of contractual rights for workers with AIDS. Employers who may make exceptions or allowances for victims of AIDS on a case-by-case basis may fear being legally bound to uphold such a standard universally, the report implies. (Chase, 1988)[102]

The more we examine the AIDS policy issues, the more complicated things appear. "Do as I say, not as I do": "Under Pentagon regulations, any applicant whose tests show that he or she carries the virus is automatically denied entry into the service." (*The New York Times*, February 7, 1988, p. 28)[103]

The vast majority of companies have no AIDS policy. But a few have rigorous policies:

Midland bank has announced its policy on AIDS in a circular to all staff. It states that where a bank employee contracts AIDS:

> "generally there will be no ground for ceasing employment or transfer to other duties but the bank will take into account any medical advice received, assess whether the individual has the ability to continue working satisfactorily, and whether continued employment is against the employee's, the bank's or the public's interest."

The company will also be distributing "AIDS packs" to its

TABLE XI

AMERICAN WAR DEAD

Revolutionary War
- Battle Deaths   6,824
- Other Deaths   18,500
-      25,324

War of 1812
- Battle Deaths   2,260
- Other Deaths   --
-      2,260

Mexican War
- Battle Deaths   1,733
- Other Deaths   11,550
-      13,283

Civil War
- North Battle Deaths   140,414
- Other Deaths   224,097
-      364,511

- South Battle Deaths   74,524
- Other Deaths   59,297
-      133,821

Total Civil War Deaths: **498,332**

Spanish - American War
- Battle Deaths   385
- Other Deaths   2,061
-      2,446

World War I
- Battle Deaths   53,513
- Other Deaths   63,195
-      116,708

World War II
- Battle Deaths   292,131
- Other Deaths   115,185
-      407,316

Korean War
- Battle Deaths   33,629
- Other Deaths   20,617
-      54,246

Vietnam War
- Battle Deaths   47,321
- Other Deaths   10,700
-      58,021

Compiled from the 1988 World Almanac by Dr. Browning

branches. These contain plastic gloves, aprons and bags to be used by staff if they need to mop up blood or other body fluids. (*Personnel Management*, August, 1987)[104]

The legal side of AIDS policy issues is complicated by other considerations that first appear to be totally unrelated to AIDS:

> In an eight-month period last year, federal appeals courts struck down city and state affirmative-action programs in San Francisco, Richmond, Va., and Michigan. All three rulings were written by judges appointed by President Reagan.
>
> Long after Mr. Reagan leaves office, his legacy will be felt in the nation's federal courtrooms. He has appointed an unprecedented 334 federal judges, 45% of the total. These judges are transforming the federal courts. . . .
>
> . . . Claims that employers or local governments discriminate based on race, sex or age become tougher to win. (Wermiel, 1987)[105]

Other court cases are examining other types of discrimination:

> The Supreme Court will hear arguments tomorrow on the jobs-discrimination case that could force managers to provide rigid justifications for subjective hiring and promotion decisions. [Clara B. Watson vs. Fort Worth Bank & Trust] (Reibstein, 1988)[106]

That is not even the end of the problems:

> Alan Tuffin, general secretary of the Union of Communication Workers and chair of the TUC's Social Insurance and Welfare Committee, stressed the need for joint involvement and action on AIDS by employers and unions.
>
> He said that he had been disappointed with employers' lack of consultation with trade unions, with a recent survey showing that where employers had introduced an AIDS policy, six out of 10 had been drawn up by management only teams. "Only 5 per cent had even thought of bringing trade union representatives into the process," continued Tuffin.

"Frankly, that is unacceptable." (*Personnel Management,* August 1987, p. 8)[107]

Employers and employees, AIDS victims and other members of society need to tackle our wide ranging problems together. This is not either/or; it is we who are economically at stake. No one will be served if any special interest group - whomever they might be - is served.

Not only business company policies but also all other AIDS policies need to be publicly addressed by everyone. Policies usually involve rights and responsibilities, and everyone's rights, including our right to life, are involved as are our responsibilities.

CONCLUSION

In the myriad of AIDS discussions that we have read, many writers have talked about the rights of AIDS victims. However, few of those writers have also discussed the obligations of AIDS victims.

AIDS victims are not separate and apart from the rest of our economic system. They have been and are wage earners contributing to our economy. As we have also repeatedly seen, those AIDS victims have made, are presently making, and will continue to make enormous economic demands on our economy.

AIDS victims are part of our social and economic population. They are members of our United States citizenry. As such, they have responsibilities and obligations just as all other citizens.

As decisions are made regarding AIDS, AIDS victims should be part of the population making those decisions. At every level, from families and business to national levels, AIDS victims need to be included. And they and everyone else making decisions need to include not only choices that favor AIDS victims but also choices that serve our entire nation.

"Bleeding hearts" who think only of short term, immediate consequences can destroy everyone's long-term good - AIDS victims' as well as everyone else's good. If short-term demands are met that undermine long-term social and economic needs, the reaction against AIDS victims will be disastrous.

As we have briefly discussed in "Medicare," general medical care costs are tremendously increasing nationally. Far more complicated and sophisticated medical technology has made life extension possible in ways never before seen. However, that same medical technology and the expertise it requires have also greatly increased medical costs in many instances.

AIDS medical treatment costs will greatly increase the already high costs of medical care. AIDS victims and all of us need to be cognizant of those combined costs. Increasingly, choices will have to be made regarding allocation of our national economic resources.

We will not be faced with an either-or choice. AIDS victims are part of our citizenry. Many other groups within the United States also require tax supported medical care. As a nation we are socially obliged to care for all.

But some hard choices will have to be made regarding who gets what. How much national economic support for medical care is available? How will that national economic support get allocated?

As AIDS cases increase and tax supported medical costs increase, we need to remember that ultimately we must examine nationally supported medical costs, not just AIDS medical costs. As contributing members of our vital country, AIDS victims need also to remember their obligations and responsibilities to the rest of their nation - all of us.

If those issues are forgotten and/or ignored, present and future ARC and AIDS victims will experience a national backlash such as never before seen in this country. For their own safety and well being now and in the future, AIDS victims must address those issues too. It will probably be far better for them in the long run if they begin by making some of the hard choices related to AIDS now.

The United States has never had any pogroms. We need to make pertinent choices concerning future economic overloads and avoid the possibility of future pogroms.

To give our readers some comparative basis for better understanding the enormous consequences of AIDS on our society, we offer you the information in Table XII on the following page.

As long as we focus on AIDS victims rather than the AIDS virus, we will confuse our own analyses. Particularly because AIDS originally came to be associated with homosexuals and drug addicts, the American public initially developed some unconscious prejudices against AIDS anything. Sexual issues, dereliction, and outright fear combined to color our opinions even before we had adequate information about AIDS.

Awareness of some of our own unconscious prejudices can help us analyze the real health and life threats the AIDS virus presents.

TABLE XII

AIDS INFECTIONS IN THE UNITED STATES & UNITED KINGDOM

United States

Year	New infections	Total infections
1978	4,132	4,132
1979	15,108	19,240
1980	67,350	86,590
1981	263,482	350,072
1982	751,897	1,101,969
1983	714,901	1,816,870
1984	669,596	2,486,466

United Kingdom

Year	New infections*	Total infections
1981	826	826
1982	9,306	10,132
1983	14,412	24,544
1984	61,098	85,642
1985	23,646	109,288

*Note that UK infections are derived from case notifications. This may cause small year-on-year anomalies in infection rates. (Rees, 1987)

That awareness can also help us analyze the present and future economic consequences of AIDS.

All of us need to begin to think in terms such as these.

1. AIDS Virus
2. AIDS Viral Transmission
3. Population Decline
4. Productivity Decline
5. AIDS Health Care
6. AIDS Deaths
7. Employers' Costs
8. City, State, & National AIDS Costs
9. AIDS Victims' Dependents' Support
10. AIDS Victims' Support
11. AIDS Health Care Costs
12. AIDS Health Care

Only by controlling our reactive emotional responses will we come to some rational decisions regarding all aspects of AIDS. We all need to stop thinking in terms of "them or us." We also need to stop thinking about AIDS as a homosexuals' and/or drug addicts' disease. The African experience has already proven that AIDS is a non-class, heterosexual disease. The evidence is in!

We need to examine our unreasonable fears now. Irrational fears could progressively create social havoc as we have never seen before. Witch burnings of the past would be nothing compared to what we could see.

Dr. Browning's description of the social terror that Jews have faced throughout the centuries would be far closer to what we could see with AIDS in the future. Convinced irrational men can be just as deadly as rational, committed men fighting for a worthy cause.

Panic combined with prejudice provide the darkroom for negatives to develop.

It is time for the morality debate to end. The health risk facts are in, and those facts are rather conclusive: AIDS is a highly contagious, sexually transmitted disease. Apparently, it does not matter what someone morally believes. We have never known anyone who was protected from a highly contagious virus by belief or a lack of some belief. It is avoidance of any highly contagious virus that counts.

AIDS IS A HIGHLY CONTAGIOUS VIRUS. . . . or as Surgeon General Koop has declared: A ". . . dangerous contagious disease."

Need we say more?

PART II:
THE SCIENCE OF AIDS

MAN

Man has, for a very long while, attempted to gain control of his environment or, if that was not possible, learn to cope with it.

A rock, held in the hand, was a slight advantage. There was always a possibility that something could be turned to human advantage by hitting it with something harder than the hand. Then, if the rock were chipped away to make a stone axe, a person could effectively have a tooth at the end of his arm. That was a definite advantage, because the human could engage the adversary at a greater distance than the adversary could engage the human.

And so it has gone through the Stone Age, the Bronze Age, the Iron Age, the Industrial Revolution, and up to the present - whatever the present might be called. Man has kept improving his advantage step by step, tool by tool, skill by skill, discipline by discipline, over his competition - which is all the other life forms. Now he stands alone as the longest lived and winner in any major contest with almost all other species. The only exceptions are certain lethal diseases.

To compare Man with the other forms, I assembled data from the *Handbook of Biological Data*.

ANIMAL	WEIGHT (Lb.)	AV. LIFE SPAN	CALCU-LATED	DEVN. FROM CALCULATED
Chipmunk	.154	2.5	-0.17	+2.67
Raccoon	4.84	4	7.23	-2.39
Agouti	5.72	6	7.62	-1.91
Monkey (Rhesus)	7.48	15	8.17	+6.83
Coyote	18.7	9	10.16	-1.16
Cheetah	46.2	6	12.09	-6.09
Wolf	48.4	12	12.19	-0.19
Leopard	105.6	14	13.87	+0.13
Chimpanzee	114.4	15-20	14.07	+0.93 to 5.93
Hyena	136.4	12	14.42	-2.42
Swine	224.4	16	15.51	+0.49
Bear (Grizzly)	308	20	16.15	+3.85
Ass (Wild)	330	14.6	16.35	-1.75
Tiger	352	11	16.50	-5.50
Buffalo (Afr.)	1540	10	19.67	-9.67
Giraffe	2640	14	20.81	-6.81
Hippopotamus	2970	40	21.06	+18.93
Elephant (Afr.)	14520	24	24.48	-0.48
Man (Ancient)	100	about 20	13.5	+6.5
Man (Modern), Worldwide	150	50	14.62	+35.38

WEIGHT AND LIFE SPANS OF VARIOUS ANIMALS AND MAN

(*Handbook of Biological Data*, Spector, ed., 1956)[1]

FIGURE 1

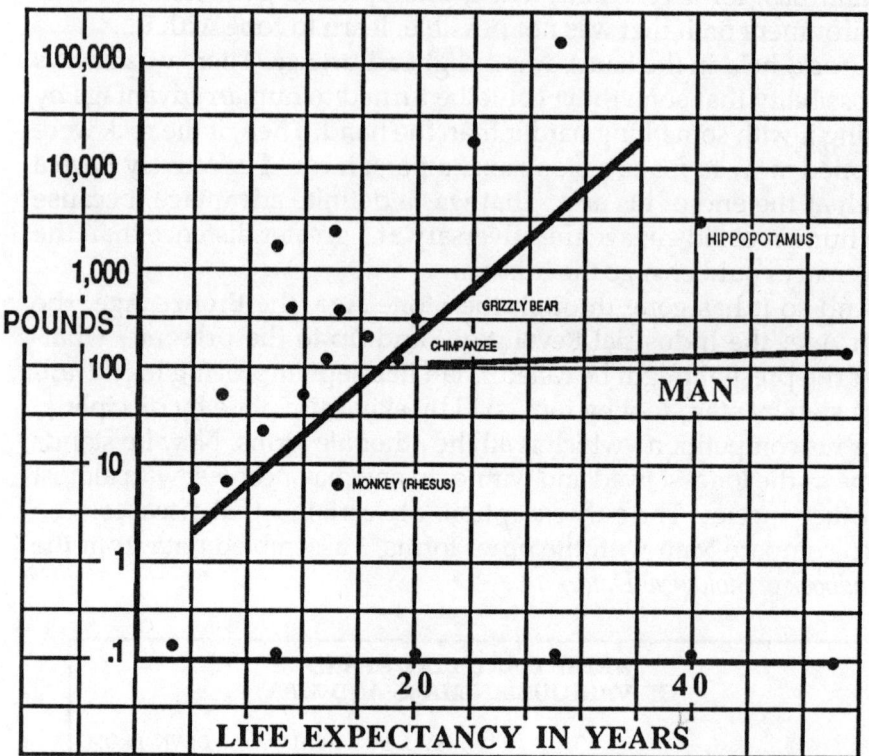

[Graph: Pounds (log scale, .1 to 100,000) vs. Life Expectancy in Years. Data points labeled HIPPOPOTAMUS, GRIZZLY BEAR, CHIMPANZEE, MAN, MONKEY (RHESUS).]

An obvious relationship exists. The line drawn through the data points is the mean slope - the relationship between weight in pounds and life expectancy.

Man has clearly broken free of the pack (See Figure 1). His natural place in the pack is at a life expectancy of about 20 years. He has domesticated plants and animals to have food available; he cooks his food to get rid of the germs (rare meat is a luxury that he can indulge in, if he is sure that there are no germs); he also has developed shelter, clothing, medicine, and insurance (in the form of family, or extended family). In fact he has laboriously gone farther and farther from the animals in nature.

The hippopotamus has specialized in the extreme in return for extended life expectancy. The Grizzly bear probably earns his extra 4.85 years - but has a limited range, and an even more limited social life.

One can assume that the Chimpanzee and the Rhesus Monkey use their brains to advantage.

But it is Man that has triumphed - with the greatest brain-to-body-surface-ratio (i.e., "intelligence") in the animal world; the best legs in the animal kingdom (Man can walk any other land animal to death.); and with his "tooth" at the end of his arm, or even further away.

Man has the least environmental inhibitions:

He lives from sea-level to high-mountains.

He lives from rain-forest to shifting-sand in the desert.

He lives from the equator to the pole.

He may burrow in rock (Gibraltar) or live on the water all his life (house boats on the Yellow River).

This gentlest and most ferocious of all creatures, Man, has learned to cope with whatever Nature has thrown at him for a million years. Given that track record, it is an article of faith that he will learn to cope with AIDS as well.

In the following pages, we will describe this current pandemic, its primary and secondary effects, and will make suggestions as to how Man can cope.

THE AFFLICTION

This SECTION deals with the nature, history, and technical aspects of the acquired immune deficiency syndrome (AIDS).

There is no appropriate time to make this report other than now. We did not know when AIDS (or as it is now called: HIV - human immunodeficiency virus) began; we do not know whether or when a cure will be found - certainly it would be at some future date as opposed to now; we do not know when the worst of the pandemic will pass (it has long since surpassed epidemic proportions); we have no idea when all of the facts will be known.

So we have elected to tell the truth as we know it (or come to know it by a search of the literature) now. We will attempt diligently to leave moral, emotional, and ethical judgements to others.

Browning has 268 reference articles before him at the beginning of this writing effort, ranging from: Scientific, medical and popular science journals, scientific article preprints, popular magazines, and newspaper and news magazine articles.

We will conjecture on future events: Scientific, medical, sociological and economic.

WHAT IS AIDS

> ... had "no choice" but to designate HIV infection (AIDS) as "a dangerous contagious disease."
> (Okie, 1978)[2]
> Dr. C. Everett Koop
> U.S. Surgeon General
> Head, Public Health Service

AIDS is a communicable, infectious condition which causes the infected human to exhibit the Acquired Immune Deficiency Syndrome. People knew about immune deficiencies.

A boy in Houston was born with an immune deficiency. He lived in a sterile plastic bubble in his home for about 12 years. Then when illness forced him out for medical treatment, he died shortly thereafter under attack from the real, unsterile world. The inherited condition was not transmitted.

People who receive organ transplants must have their immunity destroyed, else they "reject" the organ which was intended to save their lives. Unless their immunity is destroyed, they die along with the rejected organ. The immune deficient survivors do not transmit their induced condition.

PHASE I

But AIDS is different. It is transmissible.

It is noteworthy in that it is almost universally lethal. For example, according to the *British Medical Journal* - of cases reported as of 15 April 1987 in Great Britain:

TABLE I

YEAR DIAGNOSED: PER CENT OF FATALITIES

1982-1983	:	100
1984	:	83
1985	:	63
1986	:	43

(Adler, 1987)[3]

This being 1987, Great Britain has had no survivors for as long as 4 years. Each year will become 100% in its turn.

There are (as of 6 September 1987) 23 AIDS-diagnosed patients enrolled in a Long-Term Survivor Study recently launched at the Center for Disease Control in Atlanta. The earliest of these was originally diagnosed with AIDS in 1982.

It is incorrect to say that the disease is 100% fatal. To be sure, only 23 out of about 44,000 (AIDS Weekly Surveillance Report, U.S., 1987)[4] have survived up to 5 years, but it is something to hope for. (Japenga, 1987)[5]

The only disease that has ever occurred that competed with AIDS in deadliness was the pneumonic form of plague, with a mortality rate of 99.99%. (Boehm, et al., eds., 1983)[6]

It is rumored that a U.S. CDC (Center for Disease Control, Atlanta) researcher has amended the survival figures to only 2% beyond three years after diagnosis.

In the case of the longest lived AIDS patient, according to the *Los Angeles Times*, there is a scientific answer to the how-do-you-do-it question.

Dr. Jay A. Levy, professor of medicine at UC San Francisco Medical Center, has found a "subset" of lymphocytes (white blood cells) in Turner's blood that seem to act as suppressor cells. When Levy grows them in the laboratory, the AIDS virus multiplies. When he returns them to Turner's blood, the virus becomes inactive again. (Japenga, 1987)[5]

Indeed, according to doctors at the Massachusetts General Hospital, there is a newly discovered type of killer cell, called cytotoxic T lymphocytes, that seeks out the AIDS virus and destroys it. That may explain why some infected people go on to develop the disease while others do not. (UPI, 1987)[7]; (Special to *The New York Times*, 1987)[8]

AIDS was originally defined by the Center for Disease Control in America (Atlanta, GA - Ed.) as occurring in a person (a) with a reliably diagnosed disease that is at least moderately indicative of an underlying cellular immune deficiency - for example, Kaposi's sarcoma in a patient aged less than 60 years or an opportunistic infection; and (b) who has no known cause of cellular immune deficiency or any other cause of reduced resistance reported to be associated with the disease. (Adler, 1987)[3]

A subsequent definition of the disease somewhat broadened the definition. (Council of State and Territorial Epidemiologists, CDC, [Aug.] 1987)[9] New definitions add AIDS encephalopathy, the HIV wasting syndrome and the presumptive diagnosis of indicator disease to the previous definition. (Von Reyn and Mann, [Dec.] 1987)[10]

TABLE II

Human T lymphotropic virus type III (HTLV III)
Lymphadenopathy associated virus (LAV)
AIDS related/associated virus (ARV)
Human immunodeficiency virus (HIV)

Now

Acquired Immune Deficiency Syndrome (AIDS)

Considering the incredible fatality rate of AIDS, a concentrated scientific effort has been mounted that has only two precedents: The development of the atomic bomb, and the rocket to the moon, both of which were conceptually simple.

> A virus was isolated from AIDS patients "... by Barre-Sinoussi, Montagnier, and colleagues at the Institute Pasteur, Paris, in 1983, and given the name lymphadenopathy ('swollen glands') associated virus (LAV). In 1984 Popovic, Gallo, and coworkers described the development of cell lines permanently and productively infected with another AIDS virus isolate . . ." (Mortimer, 1987)[11]

According to Gallo, he and his coworkers in late 1982 and continuing throughout 1983 found preliminary evidence of the AIDS retrovirus. (Gallo, 1987)[12] I do not know which will ultimately get the credit for the discovery of the AIDS virus; but their agents will share the derived cash, according to the agreement worked out by the French and U.S. Presidents.

AIDS Antibodies Test

In 1984 a test was developed then marketed in 1985 to detect antibodies to HIV. That is what is commonly used to test a person for AIDS. It does not! It tests for the antibodies developed by the body against AIDS. (Gallo, 1987)[12] It takes time for the antibodies to develop. According to a review paper, the disease "may occur as early as one week after infection and usually precedes seroconversion, which commonly occurs between 6 to 12 weeks after infection but may take as long as 8 months." (Piot and Colebunders, 1987)[13]

Indeed, a Finnish study showed that some people do not test positive for more than a year after infection.

The Finnish scientists studied 235 homosexual or bisexual men and two women for up to three years. Of about 30 men who ultimately were found to be virus carriers, five developed antibodies latently.

The scientists, knowing who had produced the HIV antibodies, (i.e., had tested positive for them) went back to the blood samples that had been saved. They tested for the actual virus (a much more expensive test than the $5.00 antibody test) and found that five of their test people carried the actual virus 11 to 14 months earlier than their antibody (+) test.

In conclusion, "the antibodies detected by commonly used tests may not appear for as long as a year or more in 10 to 20 percent of gay men who were infected through sexual contact." (Kolata, 1987)[14]

The scientists do not conclude it, but it is reasonable to believe that these men with enough virus to produce the antibody reaction were probably contagious during at least some part of their latency period, though they had not yet tested positive.

Still another reference from the insurance industry states that "... the recent discovery that current antibody tests may not show signs of HIV exposure for up to 23 months. This could lead to problems in underwriting, he [Chuffart] said." (*National Underwriter*, 1987)[15]

In addition to the latency statistic, there is a period of dormancy. The AIDS virus may lie dormant an average of eight years before causing disease in adults infected by blood transfusions, a new study suggests.

This study extrapolated from "... data on 297 people who received tainted blood or blood products between April 1978 and February 1986 and who were diagnosed with AIDS between January 1982 and June 1986."

The estimated average dormant periods were 1.97 years for children up to age 4 at the time of infection, 8.23 years for people aged 5 to 59 years, and 5.5 years for people 60 and older. (Associated Press, 1987)[16]

HIV has been isolated from semen, cervical secretions, lymphocytes (of which pus is an example), cell free plasma, cerebrospinal fluid, tears, saliva, urine, and breast milk.

Since the concentration of virus varies considerably, it does not follow automatically that all of these transmit AIDS.

Particularly infectious are semen, blood, and possibly cervical secretions.

TABLE III
AIDS TRANSMISSION MODES

Proven common modes of transmission are:

Sexual intercourse............-Anal and vaginal

Contaminated needles......-Intravenous drug abusers
-Needlestick injuries
-Injections

Transfusions....................-Blood
-Plasma
-Blood products

Mother to child...............-In utero
-At birth
-Breast milk (Associated Press, 1987)

Organ/tissue transplants...-Kidneys
-Skin
-Bone Marrow
-Cornea
-Heart/valves
-Tendons
-Etc.

There is no well documented evidence (as of 25 April 1987) that virus is spread by: Saliva, casual or social contact, simple health care (barring needlestick or other injury), mosquitos, lice, bed bugs, in swimming pools, or by sharing cups, eating or cooking utensils, or toilets and air space shared with an infected individual. Hence, HIV infections and AIDS are not contagious. (From the *British Medical Journal*)[3]

Despite this attitude on the part of certain medical people, Dr. C. E. Koop, the U.S. Surgeon General and head of the Public Health Service, said he had "no choice" but to designate HIV infection as "a dangerous contagious disease."[2]

The rules accompanying this designation amend the list, substituting "HIV infection" for AIDS. To be infected with the virus is "HIV infection," whereas the actual disease is AIDS.

Unknown Transmission Modes

There is a Reuters report out of Chicago "that the federal government has reported increased concern for the transmission of deadly disease from men with hemophilia to their sexual partners and children."

"The report by the Centers for Disease Control (CDC) said 69 percent of children of hemophiliac fathers and mothers *who have tested positive for the AIDS virus* will also test positive for the virus." (Reuters, 1987)[18] [Browning underline] If this report stands the test of time, the case for transmission by "casual or social" contact will have been established. Indeed, *Facts on File* (1986) reports that the September 20 issue of the British Medical Journal *Lancet* tells of a German boy 3-years-old who had AIDS from a blood transfusion. His older brother caught AIDS from the younger brother. There is no proof of mechanism. (*Facts on File*, 1986)[19]

An article by George Dunea, Cook County Hospital, Chicago, IL, in the *British Medical Journal* discusses the ". . . case of a Methodist bishop in Texas, who had led an unimpeachable life but had worked with AIDS victims." He caught AIDS - UNACCOUNTABLY. (Dunea, 1987)[20]

By March 1985, (when screening became available), 92 to 95 percent of the 10,000 people in the U.S. with classical hemophilia had been infected. (Latz Griffin, 1987)[21] There are estimates that 10% to 100% of those infected will get AIDS.

In the process of diagnosis, doctors look for the following diseases as at least moderately indicative of underlying cellular immune deficiency. (See Table IV)

A different aspect of AIDS is that, though the aerosol produced by coughing may not transmit AIDS itself (and that is not for sure), such a disease as tuberculosis can become very virile in an AIDS patient. (Millar, 1987)[22] There was the case of the AIDS patient with tuberculosis who gave tuberculosis - not AIDS - to the eight members of the attendant nursing staff.

The clinical manifestations of the acute HIV seroconversion include a glandular fever like illness, encephalopathy, meningitis, myelopathy, or neuropathy. (Mindel, 1987)[23] [Note that these symptoms concentrate on neurological centers - that is one of the outstanding characteristics of AIDS.]

TABLE IV
AIDS RELATED DISEASES

Protozoa and helminthic:
Cryptosporidiosis and Isosporiasis	Diarrhoea for more than 1 month
Pneumocystis carinii	Pneumonia
Strongyloidosis	Pneumonia, Central Nervous Sys. or disseminated
Toxoplasmosis	Pneumonia or Central Nervous System (CNS)

Fungal:
Aspergillosis	CNS or disseminated
Candidiasis	Oesophageal or broncho-pulmonary
Cryptococosis	Pulmonary, CNS, or disseminated
Histoplasmosis	Disseminated

Bacterial:
"Atypical" mycobacteriosis	(Species other than tuberculosis or lepra) disseminated

Viral:
Cytomegalovirus	Lung, gut, or CNS
Herpes simplex virus	Severe mucocutaneous disease more than 1 month, pulmonary, gut or disseminated
Progressive multifocal leucoencephalopathy	

Cancer:
Kaposi's sarcoma	No age restriction
Cerebral lymphoma	
Non-Hodgkin's lymphoma	Diffuse, undifferentiated, and of B cell or unknown phenotype
Lymphoreticular malignancy	More than 3 months after

Others:
Chronic lymphoid interstitial pneumonitis in child under 13

from the *British Medical Journal*

One disease - Kaposi's sarcoma - became a diagnostic condition for AIDS because it is so unusual:

TABLE V
KAPOSI'S SARCOMA

Clinical groups of patients with Kaposi's sarcoma:

1. "Classical": Elderly, predominantly male, Jewish, or east European
2. African (various types)
3. Patients receiving immunosuppressive treatment
4. AIDS related

Kaposi's sarcoma is 10:1 male; rare multicentric vascular tumors, usually in the legs of elderly patients.

In Africa, particularly parts of sub-Saharan Africa, Kaposi's sarcoma has been endemic for many years, being like that in elderly Jewish men and a form that predominantly affects the lymph nodes in infants and young children. One variety attacks young adults.

A third variety of non-AIDS Kaposi's sarcoma occurs in patients receiving immunosuppressive therapy associated with organ transplants, especially renal (kidney) transplants.

In the case of AIDS-related Kaposi's sarcoma, lesions are usually multiple, often progress rapidly, and may affect practically any area of the skin or internal organs.

The tumors often begin as small flat dusky red or violet areas of skin discoloration, progressing in weeks or months to raised painless firm nodules and plaques. (Smith and Spittle, 1987)[24]

Gastrointestinal endoscopy at the time the condition appears shows positive for Kaposi's sarcoma in about 40% of the patients. Examination at death shows it in more than 70%. (Weller, 1987)[25]

The multicentric characteristic is a puzzle. That means that many nodules show up, with none of them being identifiable as to its origin. In ordinary cancers, the appearance of the cells is usually recognizable as to its point of origin. For example, if the cancer cells look like thyroid or liver cells, you can go to those locations and find the "primary." Any operation that does not remove the primary is just marking time. But the Kaposi's sarcoma seems to have no "primary."[24]

Kaposi's sarcoma is rarely fatal in its own right. It is, however, frequently associated with malignant lymphoma, which is deadly.[24]

In some cases, it's virtually impossible to tell whether death is AIDS-related. In the case of Hodgkins disease, it's almost impossible to tell. (Arndt, 1987)[26]

In addition to cancer, Pneumocystis carinii pneumonia accounts for 85% of lung infections in AIDS. Additionally, tuberculosis is seen more commonly in patients with AIDS than in the general population.[22]

There are many symptoms of the various characteristic and opportunistic infections that accompany AIDS. I could dwell on these to the point of virtually turning the stomach of the reader. Suffice it to say that there are a great many of the most repugnant symptoms.

It has never been physically attractive to have a disease and die. But that is what people do with AIDS. Dying has never been a question - we are all going to die. However, with AIDS, one dies relatively sooner - and with more than usual unpleasantness.

AIDS and The Young

Teenagers in the U.S. have a behavioral set that is conducive to AIDS. The Washington based Center for Population Options, after extensive examinations, said one-half the boys and one-third of the girls in the nation's high schools have had sexual intercourse at an average age of sixteen. (Cimons, 1987)[27]

An estimated 200,000 teenagers have used intravenous drugs.[27]

Only one-twelfth of the sexually active teenagers use condoms.[27] ("Safe sex with condoms" will be addressed elsewhere. It's not safe!)

One million teenagers run away from home each year; an estimated 187,500 runaways become involved in illegal activities such as drug use, drug trafficking and prostitution. A total of 125,000 to 200,000 teenaged boys and girls become involved in prostitution each year.[27]

More than 1% of high school seniors report using heroin, and use is higher among dropouts.[27]

Needle use other than drugs is: Piercing ears, possibly tattooing, and illegal steroids among athletes.[27]

In conclusion, it is clear that the nation will lose most of these young people to AIDS. Most will not choose to change their morality or behavior, and those practices are known to be conducive to AIDS, which is lethal and spreading like wildfire.

The nation bears the guilt of permitting these young people to have a lethal cultural milieu. The development of antibiotics in World War

II and the introduction of the "pill" later in the decade of the 40s, with general usage in the 50s, appeared to emancipate people with regard to casual sex and its consequent diseases and pregnancies. The "do your own thing" ethic that became rampant in the 60s and the introduction of the political cliche - "human rights" - made its way to the fore in the late 1970s. This phrase - notable for its lack of reference to "obligations" - is taken as license to do as one pleases. But bacteria and viruses are unaware of the concept of "human rights."

PHASE II

In an effort to determine the degree to which AIDS is racial, ethnic and ethically related, [as initiated by CDC Director James O. Mason, M.D., in his talk to the annual meeting of the American Council of Life Insurance: Twenty five percent of those who are ill with AIDS are black and 14 percent are Hispanic, twice the makeup in the United States population. (Fisher, 1987)[28]] I did the following study:

I acquired AIDS deaths numbers by state (and DC) from a variety of publications - presumably all data collected and reported by the Center for Disease Control, for the 1985 period.

[I wish to acknowledge great assistance by my friend, Bill Valencic, who called each state for death and infection data for 1987.] (Valencic, 1987)[29]

I prefer to work with deaths, rather than cases, because I have found that deaths are more faithfully reported than any other statistic. People almost everywhere have to account for dead human bodies. Even so, many deaths are not reported as AIDS because of family sensitivities, insurance, failure to know the cause, or other important considerations. Reporting "too low" was estimated by Dr. Mason as 20% in the case of AIDS, and 10% too low in the case of AIDS deaths.[28]

In summary of the total accumulated deaths at the two reporting times approximately 23 months apart: There had been 14,385 deaths recorded as of 11/5/85, and 26,858 deaths as of about October 1987. That is a gain of 87% in 23 months, or a doubling time of approximately 25.5 months. That mature doubling time (as compared with 8.5 months in the earlier stages of the pandemic) represents the movement of the plague from the most susceptible categories such as promiscuous homosexuals and prostitutes to the somewhat less susceptible categories of contaminated needle users (intravenous drug abusers, unsterilized acupuncture needles, etc.) thence to the heterosexual non-monogamous abusers. The doubling time will slow farther to the slowest doubling time in the heterosexual monogamous population who are not intravenous drug users. They will get AIDS in the less likely ways - by social and casual contact,[19,21] and by insect vectors. (Leishman, 1987)[30]

See Figure 2 for slowing process. The indicated stability rate is about 58 months doubling time.

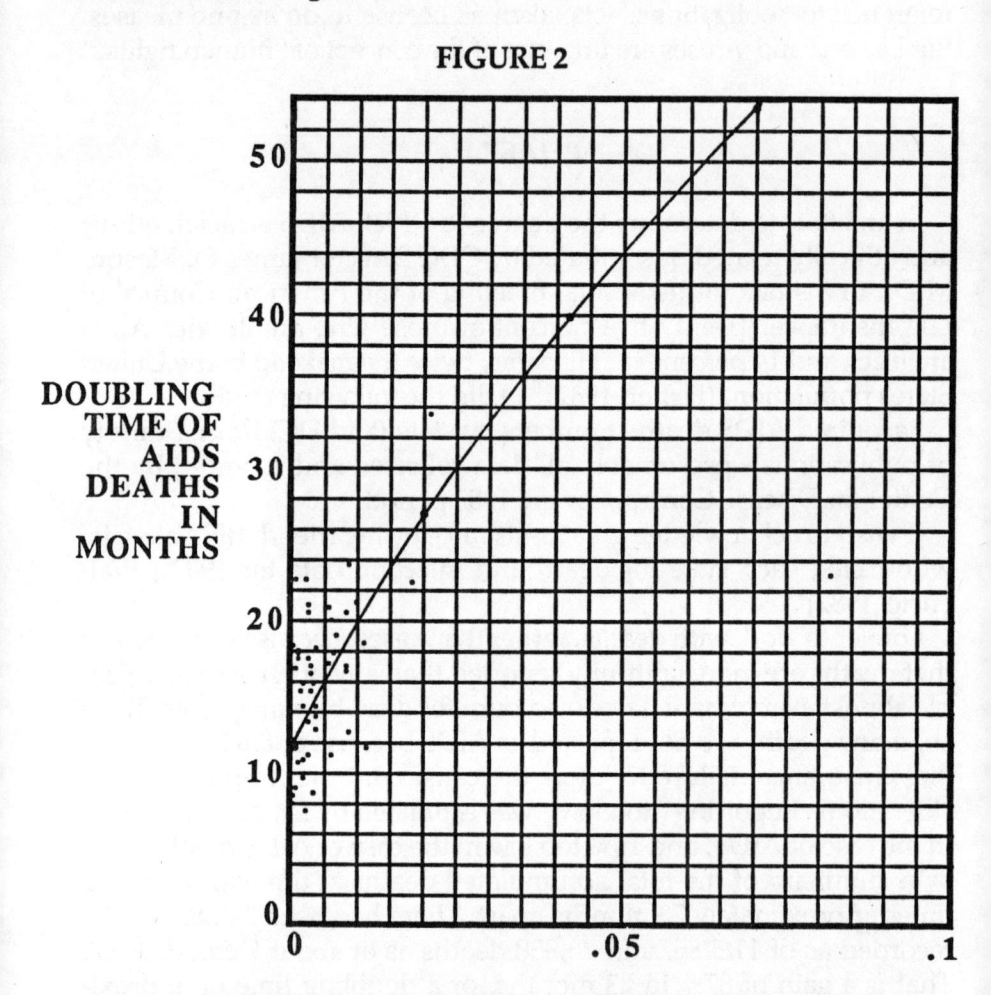

FIGURE 2

DOUBLING TIME OF AIDS DEATHS IN MONTHS

The next phase of the study involved accumulating comparable data on the States and DC covering many kinds of data.

Census data, of course, separate almost all racial and ethnic groups in the population. (*The Browning Newsletter*, Nov. 1985)[31] All of these identifiable groups, their percentages in all of the states, the percentages of AIDS deaths, and any other figures susceptible to statistical analysis were processed.

TABLE VI
DEATHS IN STATES

[1] STATES	[2] DATES	[3] DEATHS AS OF [2]	[4] DEATHS AS OF 11/5/85	[5] PER CENT OF INCREASE
ALABAMA	11/06/87	127	33	385
ALASKA	10/30/87	27	6	450
ARIZONA	11/01/87	195	73	267
ARKANSAS	11/04/87	43	17	253
CALIFORNIA	09/30/87	5398	3355	161
COLORADO	10/31/87	290	108	269
CONNECTICUT	11/04/87	339	156	217
DELAWARE	11/01/87	35	16	219
DIST. OF COLUM.	11/13/87	547	261	210
FLORIDA	11/01/87	2065	995	208
GEORGIA	11/09/87	586	230	255
HAWAII	09/14/87	88	38	232
IDAHO	11/13/87	11	0	INFINITE
ILLINOIS	11/01/87	678	307	221
INDIANA	11/06/87	141	53	266
IOWA	11/09/87	39	14	279
KANSAS	09/30/87	61	13	469
KENTUCKY	11/04/87	60	29	207
LOUISIANA	11/01/87	405	152	266
MAINE	11/05/87	29	10	290
MARYLAND	10/31/87	827	203	407
MASSACHUSETTS	11/01/87	553	276	200
MICHIGAN	11/16/87	279	95	294
MINNESOTA	11/10/87	159	48	331
MISSISSIPPI	11/13/87	56	10	560
MISSOURI	11/06/87	185	73	253
MONTANA	11/13/87	7	1	700
NEBRASKA	11/10/87	30	6	500
NEVADA	11/01/87	76	20	380
NEW HAMPSHIRE	11/01/87	26	8	325
NEW JERSEY	11/01/87	1646	888	185
NEW MEXICO	11/06/87	45	16	281
NEW YORK	09/18/87	7496	5076	148
NORTH CAROLINA	09/28/87	169	78	217
NORTH DAKOTA	11/13/87	6	0	INFINITE
OHIO	11/02/87	327	90	363
OKLAHOMA	10/30/87	95	29	328
OREGON	11/09/87	149	49	304
PENNSYLVANIA	11/13/87	756	309	245
RHODE ISLAND	11/10/87	60	23	261
SOUTH CAROLINA	08/31/87	89	44	202
SOUTH DAKOTA	11/01/87	4	1	400
TENNESSEE	10/31/87	171	24	713
TEXAS	11/06/87	1869	748	250
UTAH	11/06/87	67	24	279
VERMONT	11/09/87	12	4	300
VIRGINIA	11/05/87	297	155	192
WASHINGTON	11/10/87	366	162	226
WEST VIRGINIA	11/13/87	23	11	209
WISCONSIN	10/30/87	147	32	459
WYOMING	11/10/87	10	1	1000

Standard sources (Year Books, Almanacs, and Statistical Abstracts of the United States, for example) were used for this sweeping study[31] (*The Browning Newsletter*, Dec. 1985)[32] as well as statistical reference books. (Lamont, *et al.*, Hoffman, *et al.*, 1977)[33]

Each of the identifiable groups (by state and DC) was correlated with the percentage of AIDS deaths (by state and DC). The correlation coefficient with 50 states and DC had 49 degrees of freedom (a statistical measure), and the correlation is expressible as "degree of certainty"[33] of the relationship.

The general statement may be made from this huge study that AIDS relates to every aspect of huge population centers. Everything that occurs more in cities, inherently correlates with the percentage of AIDS deaths - which is greatest in cities. Every activity, every attitude, every criminal statistic, drug use, the higher concentration of populations of some ethnic groups or professional group - obviously correlates with AIDS deaths percentages.

TABLE VII
POPULATION GROUPINGS

1980 population per square mile
1981 chronic liver diesase and cirrhosis
1984 per cent of voters voting Democratic for President
1984 per cent of voters voting Republican for President
1983 murder rate
1983 crime rate per 100,000
1981 suicide rate

Statistics say nothing of causes, but one might be permitted the surmise that urban life is more permissive - or at least far more impersonal - than rural life. Perhaps that bears on the higher percentage of AIDS deaths in the urban environment than in the rural environment.

An example of that is the statistic that the four most populous states (CA, NY, TX, FL) have the 11% (+) rate among men from 30–39, inclusive.[15] Most of these will be lost at great social and economic loss to those states. The less populous states have nothing like that.

Valencic's number of dead[29] - 26,858 plus the estimated 10% underreporting[28] - represents a total of 230 immigrants with AIDS, (mostly Haitians and Cubans from the Mirabel boat lift of 123,000 illegal immigrants and a scattering of others) that had doubled only seven times.

Only 12 doublings of the present number of AIDS deaths will

account for about one half the population of the U.S. Current costs exceed $100,000 each, and with 120,000,000 deaths, the costs would exceed $120 trillion. At some point, the system breaks down. (Several AIDS clinics and an AIDS hospital have gone bankrupt; this is announced to be the worst year for banks in U.S. history; and the U.S. government - with its $1 + trillion budget has had to cut expenditures that it didn't want to reduce. The handwriting is on the wall.)

The significance of the pattern indicated in Figure 2 is that the doubling time may stabilize at around four years, ten months. The doubling time will become infinite (i.e., there will be no more doubling beyond one-half the population) after 12 doublings. That will intuitively be about 60 years from the present; hence the survivors will have been separated out about 2050 A.D. Around that time, I postulate that the world population will have been reduced to about one half its present number.

PHASE III
The Complexity of the AIDS Virus

> Despite the attention, most of the researchers involved in the effort to unravel the secrets of HIV and AIDS were attracted originally by an intense fascination with this virus, which engages the human immune system in a deadly, intricate duel. It is a duel that pairs two almost perfectly matched antagonists, and at times it is almost difficult to tell them apart. Given the dizzying complexity of the immune system, this duel sometimes seems as though it were being conducted in a hall of mirrors. There has never been anything else like it. (Baum, 1987)[34]

It has been determined that there are two viruses that can cause AIDS. These viruses are designated HIV-1 and HIV-2, both almost certainly originated in Africa. The first is found predominantly in Central Africa, and the latter appears more often in West Africa.

The viruses for HIV are retroviruses, in which the genetic material is ribonucleic acid (RNA) rather than desoxyribonucleic acid (DNA). That is wholly unique because the genetic stuff of the entire animal kingdom is DNA. These retroviruses carry with them an enzyme called reverse transcriptase, a polymerase that catalyzes transcription of viral RNA into double-helical DNA (the stuff of all heredity). This stuff may exist either in an unintegrated form in the infected cell, or a copy, which is called proviral DNA may be integrated into the nucleus (genome) of the infected cell, where it may lie in a latent form, or, alternatively, produce RNA resulting in new viruses. This feature of infecting a cell in such a way as to make it its own enemy is unprecedented.[34] "We have found the enemy, and he is us." Pogo.

The viruses consist of 8 genes, whose chemical composition is known in total detail, and whose functions are moderately well understood. The viruses attack a kind of white blood cell - the T4 lymphocyte - and by whatever means [i.e., the means are not understood], reduce its numbers.[34]

Humility Not Hubris

To use an analogy: We have a tremendous amount of information about, and understanding of VOLCANOS. But our knowledge and our understanding neither prevents volcanic eruptions nor loss of life. We humans must have humility, for nature is enormously greater than we.

> As Dr. Gallo said in his *Scientific American* article: "Does this terrible tale have a moral? Yes. In the past two decades one of the fondest boasts of medical science has been the conquest of infectious disease, at least in the wealthy countries of the industrialized world. The advent of retroviruses with the capacity to cause extraordinarily complex and devastating disease has exposed that claim for what it was: hubris.[12]

> But back to the immediate subject:

> These T4 cells are "responsible for the induction directly or indirectly of most, if not all, of the functions of the human immune system."[34]

In addition - the means are not completely understood - most people who are infected with AIDS suffer deterioration of the nervous system. Richard Price and others at the Memorial Sloan-Kettering Cancer Center in New York have shown that the virus caused serious dementia, or loss of mental function, in virtually all advanced cases of AIDS. Spinal cord degeneration had also been found in AIDS patients. (*Facts on File*, 1985)[35]

Scientists found a second type of body cell attacked by the AIDS virus. The cells were the so-called monocyte/macrophages found in the brain and lung. Unlike the immune system's T-cells, the brain cells "just keep pumping out more virus." The discovery offered a possible explanation for the neurological problems associated with AIDS. (*Facts on File*, 1985)[36]

Still another mechanism has been found regarding brain problems: The University of Chicago and the University of California at Los Angeles (UCLA) found that there is an interaction of a part - about 44 amino acids long - of the AIDS virus that inhibits neuroleukin. That substance is necessary for some kinds of nerve cells to grow and thrive. (Van, 1987)[37]

The U.S. Military has determined to turn down all recruits who are very high risk. That includes all homosexuals and intravenous drug users. [Presumably, they have long since decided to turn down all hemophiliacs.] They will also exclude all those that they can determine have been exposed to AIDS. (*Facts on File*, 1985)[38]

They give as reasons for their decision: The need for rapid deployment anywhere, without concern for soldier's health; the use of vaccinations that could kill an AIDS sufferer; and the need for soldiers to supply battlefield blood transfusions. Nor do they want the burden of caring for the disease.[38]

[As one who did over 4 years of military service in World War II, may I add a couple of things? That business of a high probability of dementia - which is firmly established - I would not have considered it a favor to have had someone with both dementia and a machine gun at my side. Nor would I have wanted anyone from whom I could have contracted a fatal disease as an immediate associate. There were times when burning tumbleweeds (with thorns) had to be stopped from rolling under airplanes; and I didn't need to be thinking about thorns with a fatal disease awaiting my grasp.]

In 1985, findings indicated that only 5% to 19% of those who tested positive actually contract the disease.[38] However, according to Anthony S. Fauci, director of the National Institute of Allergy & Infectious Diseases (NIAID), ". . . studies measuring immune system deterioration in HIV-infected individuals, rather than clinical manifestation of disease, suggest that up to 80% suffer some deterioration within five years of infection."

The director of the United Nations World Health Organization [Mahler] announced 20 November 1985 a top priority drive against AIDS. He called the spread of the deadly disease a "health disaster of pandemic proportions" and said he could "not imagine a worse health problem in this century."

According to Dr. Halfdan Mahler, the director, there would be 500,000 to 3.5 million cases of AIDS by 1990. Another 100 million people might be infected with the chief AIDS virus, but be free of the disease's debilitating symptoms." (*Facts on File*, 1986)[39]

Like numbers were obtained by the General Accounting Office from the World Health Organization for Senator Jesse Helms, ranking Republican on the Senate Foreign Relations Committee, and reported to the press. (Associated Press, 1987)

Inasmuch as the consensus is that about 80% of the infected will die of the disease, that implies that 80,000,000 will die as of the infection count of 1990 (perhaps a third of that per year). Keep in mind that the world's population increases at 75,000,000 per year, and you will see that the world's population will soon quit growing, and start down, as a result of AIDS.

The worst news was released from the AIDS data bank at Los Alamos National Laboratory. (Spice, 2 September 1987)[41]; (Rensberger, 1987)[42] That data bank was established in January 1987 as a computerized clearinghouse for research on the genetic makeup of the AIDS virus. It is an outgrowth of Los Alamos' GenBank which does the same thing regarding human gene research. (Spice, 14 September 1987)[43]

They have found that the mutation rate of the AIDS virus is five times that of influenza; 1% per year, overall; and 1.5% for the gene for the envelope that surrounds it.[43]

HIV-1 and HIV-2 differ by 40 to 60%. It would have taken only 40 years for the two to have evolved far enough that a single test would not have detected both.[43]

One decedent was found to have harbored 58 different versions of the virus; the average decedent carried more than two.[43]

The clinical expression of infection with the human immunodeficiency virus (HIV) appears increasingly complex.[13]

AIDS is more complicated than we thought - even in our darkest moments; and COMPLICATION OF THE DISEASE, PER SE, IS OUR ENEMY.

PHASE IV

In addition to all of the things that we don't know, there are things that we do know that we don't understand.

1. A rare form of arthritis known as Reiter's Syndrome which occurred in 1 to 2% of the population occurs much more often, now, in people who carry the AIDS virus. (Kolata, 1987)[14]

2. Doctors are seeing many more psoriasis cases now because of AIDS.[44]

3. Women who test positive for the AIDS antibodies have twins about eight times more frequently than those who do not test positive. (Hines, 1987)[45]

4. Often, when twins are born to AIDS infected mothers, one turns out to have the disease and the other does not.[45]

CONCLUSIONS

AIDS is "a dangerous contagious disease." There is hard data to prove that it has been transmitted by:

1. Transfusion of contaminated blood;
2. Shared, unsterilized hypodermic needles;
3. Unsterilized acupuncture needles; (Gargan, 1987)
4. Homosexual sex;
5. Heterosexual sex;
6. Prostitutes;
7. Birth from a mother who tests (+);
8. Mother's milk from a mother who tests (+);
9. Normal parent/children relationships up to age five;
10. Normal parent/children relationships involving infected hemophiliac parents; and
11. A three-year-old boy to his brother

It may be transmitted by:

12. Blood sucking insects;
13. Kissing;

14. Biting (children); and

15. Other lesser forms of contact.

No one can truthfully assert that such forms of transmission cannot occur. Science cannot prove a negative. The only truthful assertion is that the probability of the second class of possible transmission methods is smaller than the first.

The more permissive a society, the higher the percentage of AIDS deaths. Population wide statistics show that the people with the higher risk of AIDS deaths are those in more dense populations in the United States.

The forced conclusion is that the more permissive a society is, the higher will be the percentage of AIDS deaths. In the end, it will all work out. ONLY THE SURVIVORS GET TO TEACH ETHICS.

These are very hard statistical facts and cannot be modified by anybody's opinion; whatever humanitarian, religious, racial, ethnic or financial basis might be used as a rationale for a contrary opinion. Facts are facts.

THE HISTORY OF AIDS

While it is no longer certain that the AIDS virus got its start in Africa, many researchers, such as Reinhard Kurth, a virologist at the Paul Erlich Institute in Frankfurt, still believe in an African origin. He believes that the malady has long existed as a "village disease" in isolated areas. (*World Press Review*, February, 1987)[47]

In Uganda, where AIDS is known as "slim disease" because of its victims' wasted bodies, it was not until 1982 that enough people died of it for others to take notice. "It was a typical smugglers' disease," says Jack Jagwe of the Ministry of Health in Kampala. "The people were always traveling, and carried the virus from one brothel or bar to the next."[47]

The timing of the origin of AIDS virus can be inferred from the mutation rate and the difference between strains. The AIDS virus is altering its genetic code by at least 1 per cent per year. HIV-1 and HIV-2, or East and West Africa, respectively, differ genetically by 40 to 60 per cent. It took about 40 years for HIV-1 and HIV-2 to diverge genetically enough that a single type of blood test would be unable to detect both. As the disease spreads, the mutation rate seems to be rising, and some of the variants of HIV-1 may already be beyond the bounds of detection.[43]

That puts the virus at least 40 years before a man in Kinshasa, Zaire, had his blood drawn and saved in 1959. Many years later, that saved blood was shown to have AIDS. He had to have had the virus at least a year, probably 2 years. He thus acquired AIDS no later than 1958. (*Chicago Tribune*, 25 October 1987)[48] That puts the beginning of the spread of AIDS from East to West Africa no later than 1917–18. In turn, the disease existed an indeterminate length of time in East Africa before its travels began.

About Christmas of 1958, a man who had been in the British Navy from 1955–57, and who had suffered the symptoms of Kaposi's sarcoma and other symptoms for two years, presented himself to the Royal Infirmary. He died in August of 1959 of pneumocystis carinii pneumonia (PCP).[48]

He obviously - in retrospect - had had AIDS since the end of 1956, and - in his Navy travels - circumstantially seems to have caught it early in 1956. Although he died of PCP and seemed to have had Kaposi's sarcoma, the doctors could find no immune deficiency. (Crewdson, 1987)[49]

In February 1967, a Black boy, 14 years of age, became sick in St. Louis. He died at 16 years of age in May 1969. The circumstances of his death were so strange that tissues were saved for subsequent study. He had a severe case of Chlamydia. For nearly two years, his lower legs and genitals (genital edema and severe proctitis) had been swollen (i.e., since 1966 when he was 13). He had a rampant case of Kaposi's sarcoma; severe in the rectal and anal areas - almost guaranteeing that he had been a homosexual prostitute. He had a severe immune deficiency.[48,49]

It is a story without a beginning or an end. It is not known whom he got it from, nor to whom he gave it. It simply says that tragedy established AIDS in or near St. Louis in 1966.

In 1979, a white male homosexual, 44, was diagnosed with Kaposi's sarcoma in New York City. The patient is believed to be the first victim of what will come to be known as Acquired Immunodeficiency Syndrome.[48]

> The first cases of AIDS in Uganda were suspected during the last quarter of 1982 when several businessmen died at Kasensero, an isolated small fishing village on Lake Victoria.

Since the disease first appeared in 1982, it has spread fast. The disease is spreading eastward along the Trans-African Highway, which handles considerable human traffic and interaction; 33% of long-distance truck drivers are infected. Civil disturbance that leads to the displacement of large adult populations is also a factor to be considered in the further spread of the disease. (Okware, 1987)[50]

In 1983, I wrote in my Newsletter as follows:

AIDS continues to occupy an intense limelight. The European regional office of the World Health Organization agreed to set up a centre equivalent to the Centers of Disease Control at Atlanta. The disease continues to increase at an exponential rate both in Europe and in the U.S., though with only about 10% as many cases in Europe as in the U.S.

The African connection seems strong, inasmuch as the major epidemics in Europe are in France and Belgium, the two countries with the strongest ties to Africa. In the Western Hemisphere, it has been suggested that Cubans returning from the wars in Africa (then their illegal immigration into the U.S., with up to one third of the emigres alleged to be homosexuals) brought, along with the Haitians, AIDS into the U.S. It has also been turned up as a report that Haiti as a vacation resort provides easy access to homosexual partners. AIDS has been shown to be endemic in equatorial Africa for a long time.

Extreme promiscuity of homosexuals: (1100 sex partners in a lifetime for an AIDS case studied - against "only" 500 in a control group of healthy homosexuals). Homosexual males practice a degree of promiscuity and intensity unknown between heterosexuals, and some doctors theorize that repeated exposure lies at the heart of the answer to the question: 'Why now?' " (Browning, 1983)[51]

In February 1983, according to CNN News, the number of AIDS cases was 1300. One year later, it was 3600. That made the doubling time 8.166 months. (Browning, March 1984)[52] (Compare that with the CNN News figure on January 3, 1988, number of cases - 46,000 and 1,500,000 infected in the U.S.)

The American Navy gave an aircraft carrier crew shore leave in Mombasa, Kenya. The crew was warned that tests had shown that 2/3 of the prostitutes in Mombasa tested positive for AIDS." (Browning, November 1986)[53]

A German study (reported in *Nature* on 20 November 1986) from the University of Frankfurt concluded that:

Three-quarters of those infected with the AIDS (Acquired Immune Deficiency Syndrome) virus will enter the final and fatal stages of the disease within seven years . . .

Further, they found that 377 of the 543 patients, "largely the sexual partners of the first AIDS victims to die in Frankfurt," became infected. Thus: 69% became infected, and 75% of those will die in 7 years. The product: 52% of those exposed will die in 7 years. (*Nature*, December 1986)[54]

In December 1986, it was reported that ". . . the highest rates of infection are invariably in prostitutes, with figures ranging from 27 to 88 per cent. More alarming are the figures of 10–20 per cent from blood donors and antenatal clinics, as these are not high-risk groups in Western terms.

Quin *et al.*, boldly state that the present annual incidence of infection is approximately 0.75 per cent among the general population of central and east Africa. Nor are there many random population surveys; but a 6 per cent rate of infection recorded in a neighborhood in Kinshasa, Zaire, is an indication of how serious the problem is. (*Nature*, December 1986)[55]

As of February 1987: "Six per cent of all blood samples tested in Zaire are positive," reports Peter Piot, a Belgian expert on tropical diseases. "In Kigali, the capital of Rwanda, it is 18 per cent." Another study shows that a third of all the sexually active men between 30 and 35 in Lusaka, the capital of Zambia, have the virus in their bodies.[47]

"Thirteen per cent of the newborns in a Kinshasa clinic come into the world doomed."[47]

By May 30, 1987, the *British Medical Journal* carried an article that claimed that:

About 10% of patients with the Acquired Immune Deficiency Syndrome (AIDS) present because of neurological problems, but as many as 75% have evidence of the disease of the nervous system at necropsy. The neurological manifestations of AIDS may be caused by opportunistic infections, by tumors, and by the primary neurological effects of the Human Immunodeficiency Virus (HIV). (Carne, 1987)[56]

On June 12, 1987, the proceedings were published: ". . . of a recent meeting in Washington, D.C., is that AIDS continues to spread and presents a major global health problem, but many scientific and epidemiological questions remain about transmission of the virus. . . ."

AIDS in Africa. "The information is sketchy and incomplete" says I. S. Okware of the Ministry of Health in Entebbe, Uganda. "But one thing is clear. The disease is spreading and spreading fast."

"Twenty-five per cent of AIDS patients in the United States have a history of drug abuse," says Peter Selwyn of Albert Einstein College of Medicine in Bronx, New York, who heads a study of 470 people enrolled in a methadone program in the Bronx. A total of 184, or 39%, now carry the AIDS virus; more Blacks and Hispanics are infected with HIV than Whites. (*Research News*, 1987)[57]

There were 20,000 hemophiliacs in the U.S. who were at risk for exposure to the AIDS virus prior to the availability of heat-treated clotting factor [or the antibody test for HIV infection] in 1985. 70% have antibodies to HIV and of those infected 331 have now developed AIDS.[57]

According to CDC's 22 May 1987 *Morbidity and Mortality Weekly Report*, three "health care workers" were infected. These three plus six previous are the totality of this class of "at risk" people who have AIDS, or test positive.[57]

The issue of health care workers is the only case where there is a categorical confusion. The other is a quote from *The Dallas Morning News* (September 21, 1987) [and I will not give the name of the person quoted]:

"--------------------" . . . for the National Centers for Disease Control in Atlanta, said 1,875 cases of AIDS among health care workers were reported as of July [1987]. That amounts to 5.8% of the total number of AIDS cases reported nationwide. The level of infection among health care workers - as in the general population - is approaching 1 per cent, experts say. (Rist, 1987)[58]

I do not know how these "health care workers" are categorized, but I suspect that the former are "health care workers in a formal clinical setting," whereas the latter may be anyone whose contact patients may be classed as "health care workers" - who do not have the clinical environment, nor clinical knowledge. That is the author's surmise, or attempt at reconciliation of the two sets of data, since he does not automatically attribute dishonesty to anyone.

AIDS was the leading cause of death for women aged 25 to 34 last year [1986], the second most frequent cause for those 35 to 39 and the third-ranking cause for those 20 to 24.

TABLE VIII
NEW YORK AIDS DEATHS (from NY City Dept. of Health)

DEATHS PER YEAR

YEAR	TOTAL	MALE	FEMALE	CASES DIAGNOSED
1983	425	376	49	994
1984	952	826	126	1735
1985	1663	1463	200	2750
1986	2650	2265	385	3317

AIDS continued to be the leading cause of death among men from ages 25 to 44 in the city [New York City], as has been true for the past few years. (Lambert, July 8, 1987)[59]

New Yorkers are now dying at the rate of 200 a month. (Lambert, July 12, 1987)[60]

A report written by Dr. Donald S. Burke of the Walter Reed Army Institute of Research in Washingyon and published in the *New England Journal of Medicine* (July 16, 1987) reported the following:

TABLE IX
AIDS TESTS ON 306,061 MILITARY RECRUITS--10/85-3/86

New York City	20.3 per 1000 Men	(2.03%)
	17.4 per 1000 Women	(1.74%)
San Francisco	11 per 1000 Men	(1.10%)
	10.9 per 1000 Women	(1.09%)
Washington, D.C.	10.7 per 1000 Men	(1.07%)
	7.3 per 1000 Women	(0.73%)
U.S. Total	1.5 per 1000 Recruits	(0.15%)
U.S. Military	1.65 per 1000 Military	(0.165%)
Nationwide, Overall	3.89 per 1000 Blacks	(0.389%)
	1.07 per 1000 Latinos	(0.107%)
	.88 per 1000 White	(0.088%)
	1.65 per 1000 Men	(0.165%)
	.61 per 1000 Women	(0.061%)

These are young, healthy recruits - with hemophiliacs, homosexuals and drug users being told in advance that they were unacceptable. (Associated Press, July 16, 1987)[61] (*The Washington Post*, July 16, 1987)[62] (Nelson, 1987)[63]

Dr. Jonathan Mann, an American who is director of the World Health Organization's special program on AIDS says: "The whole perspective is changing in response to fears of what will happen if we don't deal with the problem." ("AIDS: A Global Assessment"; *Los Angeles Times Supplement*, 1987)[64]

So far, 130 of the world's 160 countries have reported a total of 56,000 AIDS cases (August 9, 1987).[64]

The health care system has already been overwhelmed in Haiti and parts of Central Africa. The AIDS virus is estimated to be carried by 5–10 million as of August 9, 1987.[64]

"Sterilization of needles at the rural and urban hospitals of Uganda has broken down,. . ."[64]

> Scientists are still unsure how the AIDS virus is passed from mothers to unborn children and infants. But they estimate

that about half the babies born to carriers of the virus will contract AIDS and die before their fifth birthdays. . . .

" 'I think our second-biggest health problem may be the persons who get another disease, thinks it is AIDS and hopeless, and then dies because he didn't seek treatment,' said Yorokamu Kamacerere, the district administrator."[64]

Many articles point out that ear piercing, nose piercing (widespread in India), cuticle trimming, barber shop shaving, hair-cutting (nicking), acupuncture needles, thorns on paths where everyone goes barefoot, etc., can transmit AIDS.

In the Soviet Union, for example, newspapers only recently ran their first candid stories about the existence of prostitution, homosexuality and drug addiction. Although Valentin Pokrovsky said in an interview that homosexuals, prostitutes and drug users 'must be under permanent surveillance,' the Soviet Union has no official plans to give them periodic blood tests or examinations.[64]

Dr. Pokrovsky, president of the Soviet Academy of Medical Science said on August 17, 1987 that there are some 130 people in the Soviet Union infected with AIDS, most of them foreigners. (*Nature*, September 1987)[65]

It was well known to us who were in the U.S. Army that the Soviet Army took prostitutes wherever it went in World War II - and it seems unlikely that they have changed fundamentally. Although the Soviet Union continues its scurrilous propaganda and general misbehavior, AIDS has forced it "out of the closet" to a degree. Maybe the devastating plague will make them a member of the world community, when they perceive that survival, itself, depends upon cooperation. That would be a historic step.

Dentists have become worried since in a recent survey one out of 1231 seems to have been infected by a patient.[20]

The Minority percentage of AIDS cases is rising. (Griffin and Galvan, 1987)[66]

As the reader can see, the minorities are hardest hit by AIDS in the U.S.[66] (*Information Please Almanac*, 1988)[67] (*AIDS Weekly Surveillance Report*, CDC, October 12, 1987)[68]

TABLE X
WHITES, BLACKS, HISPANICS

RACE	RACE PER CENT POPULATION	AIDS CASES TOTAL PER CENT	PER CENT OF CASES PER PER CENT OF POPULATION
White	83.2	61	0.733
Black	11.69	25	2.139
Hispanic	6.45	14	2.170

In the high risk states such as California, Florida, New York, and Texas, it is estimated that 11 per cent of the male population between the ages of 30 and 39 have the HIV virus.[15]

Another concern is the recent discovery that current antibody tests may not show signs of HIV exposure for up to 23 months.[15] As reported before in these pages, a paper that we have been unable to obtain in *LANCET* is said to have reported that the latency period is up to 36 months. [As a biologist, I assert that it is possible to transmit the disease before testing positive for the antibody. I.B.]

DISCUSSION

The history of AIDS was quiet at the beginning but has become important to the world in the last decade. By virtue of its deadly record - with no more than 2% survival beyond 3 years - it has become one of the Great Plagues in the history of Mankind.

At first, it seemed as though it would kill everybody; then three hopeful and separate kinds of data showed up:

TABLE XI
TRANSMISSION PROBABILITY

Baby born of (+) mother (prob. of transmission)	25-50%
Any baby of (+) mother (prob. of death by 5 years)	50%
Any child of (+) hemophiliac parent (p. of (+) test)	69%

1. The University of Frankfurt study[54] that showed only 69% infection (in four years of outpatient's clinic attention) among those "largely the sexual partners of the first AIDS victims to die in Frankfurt," and only 75% of those will die in seven years; i.e., .69 X .75 - .52. That is to say: Only 52% of those persons who were exposed to the most likely way to be infected with HIV were expected to die within 7 years.

2. The August 9, 1987 *Los Angeles Times* insert entitled "AIDS: GLOBAL ASSESSMENT":[64] in the article titled: "Toll Threatens Hard-Earned Gains in Nations With Meager Resources," the quote:

"Scientists are still unsure how the AIDS virus is passed from mothers to unborn children and infants. But they estimate that about half the babies born to carriers of the virus will contract AIDS and die before their fifth birthdays." (Being born to a mother who carries HIV is certainly severe exposure.)

That does not seriously disagree with the quote: "The overall risk of HIV transmission from an infected mother to infant ranges from 25% to 50%."[10] After all, an infant has not reached its fifth birthday, and that might well bring death up to 50%.

Combine that with the statement from an insurance conference ". . . current antibody tests may not show signs of HIV exposure for up to 23 months . . ."; and that five years of age is well over 23 months, and you have the hope that about half of us are genetically immune.

3. The cumulative risk of HIV transmission to long term heterosexual partners is about 50%, although the range of risk is wide."[10]

These data make the case that the longer a parent/child relationship endures, the greater the probability that a (+) parent will infect the child. The relationship is SOCIAL, not CASUAL. The exposures are many; the level of risk at any exposure is small. There is not an aseptic relationship between parents and children. This, in turn, can be understood statistically as follows:

THE PRODUCT OF MANY SMALL PROBABILITIES IS A LARGE PROBABILITY

My explanation is as follows:

Every human inherits a system of barriers:

1. The first echelon barrier to the outside world is the epithelium. This is found in greatest resistance all over the body and in the vagina. It does not barricade if sex is homosexual, nor if sex is oral. In these latter cases, the barricade system number one has been finessed.

2. The second echelon barrier to those diseases which have arrived through the first echelon barrier from the outside world is chemical - otherwise known as the immune system. People who finesse their first barrier challenge themselves. That is done by more exotic sexual behavior, unsterile i.v. needles, contaminated blood on cuts - you know the ways!

THE FIRST BARRIER SEEMS TO STOP HALF OF AIDS INFECTIONS.

WHEN PEOPLE LEARN TO COOPERATE WITH THEIR BARRIERS, HALF SHOULD SURVIVE. UNTIL THEN, ONLY A FOURTH.

MY HOPE IS THAT ABOUT HALF OF US WILL SURVIVE.

SURVIVAL WILL BE UNEVEN RACIALLY AND ETHNICALLY, BUT MAN, HIMSELF, IS NOT AT RISK.

My reason for being hopeful is that only survivors will get to teach ethics!

COPING WITH AIDS

In my *Browning Newsletter*: Vol. 7, No. 1, 21 February 1983, I wrote:

> The inevitable pestilence of the 20th century (AIDS Acquired Immune Deficiency Syndrome) has arisen rather predictably among homosexuals and Haitians two groups who, for one reason or another, give disease a maximum chance to proliferate.
>
> Now the homosexuals, many of whom acquire income by selling their blood, insist that enquiry into their homosexuality (hence probable disease) is an intrusion into their privacy.
>
> Hence medicine, hobbled by social taboo, is the massive vector for this new "Black Plague." (Browning, February 21, 1983)[69]

Indeed, since February 1983, medical technology via blood transfusions,[20,38] dirty needles (an abuse of a medical technology),[20,27,38] injection of blood products into hemophiliacs, resulting in tens of thousands of cases of AIDS,[21] have been primary vectors for the disease. And now a Canadian probably got AIDS from an acupuncture needle in China.[46] Imagine 900,000,000 Chinese (the rural population of China) who don't believe in the germ theory and practice acupuncture.

Medicine has a long way to go to change from the problem to the answer.

A SHORT HISTORY OF PLAGUES

In the past, plagues have taken a great toll. All great plagues have had the characteristic that they defy previous methods of coping with diseases. That is a fair description of AIDS.

In 400 AD, a cycle of plagues began that reached its peak during the reign of Justinian I (527–65 AD), centering on 542–43 AD (McNeill, 1976),[70] and best estimates indicate as many as 100,000,000 died in the world. (Cornell, 1976)[71] The plague ". . . can confidently be identified as bubonic."[70] It is named after the large, hot lumps known as "bubos." "Often these bubos formed huge black welts," thus its other name: "Black Death."[70]

The earliest Chinese description of bubonic plague was in 610 AD.[70]

In 1320–21, epidemics in France were blamed on lepers as "well poisoners." They ". . . were believed to have acted at the instigation of the Jews and the Moslem King of Granada, in a great conspiracy of outcasts to destroy Christians." Hundreds of lepers were burned in France in 1322, and Jews were punished. (Tuchman, 1978)[72]

The outbreak of the bubonic plague is believed to have begun with a great famine in China between 1333 and 1337, which killed an estimated 4,000,000 people[71]: This is associated with the plague that began in 1331 and killed 9/10 of the population in Hopei Province.

In 1347, a Tatar army broke its siege because it had an outbreak of plague. The Tatars may have catapulted bodies dead of plague into the cities. In any case, the disease showed up in Italy (1347); North Africa, Spain, France, and England (1348); Germany (1348); and Scotland and Scandinavia (1350).

When the plague broke out in France, Jews were accused of being "well poisoners" with intent "to kill and destroy the whole of Christendom and have lordship all over the world." Lynchings began in France in the spring of 1348, where Jews were dragged from their houses and thrown in bonfires.[72]

In Savoy, the first formal trials were held in September 1348. Confessions were obtained ". . . according to the usual medieval method . . ." The charges were of an international Jewish conspiracy emanating from Spain, with messengers from Toledo carrying poison in little packets or in a ". . . narrow stitched leather bag . . ." with "rabbinical instructions for sprinkling the poison in wells and springs . . ."[72]

Eleven Jews were burned to death, others punished.

The governmental and Church establishments tried to protect the Jews; but the pogroms raged on.[72]

In city after city, mobs slaughtered Jews. "At Worms in March 1349, the Jewish community of 400 burned themselves to death in their own houses rather than be killed by their enemies."[72]

Most of the Jews in Western Europe were killed. The killing did not stop until the plague had passed, with a toll of 75,000,000.[6]

The unique form that most of the slaughter took was at the instigation of penitents (200 to 1000 in a group), whipping themselves with whips of hard knotted leather with little iron spikes. Some made themselves bleed very badly [like Shi'ite Moslems in Iran today]. [Ladies dabbled their clothing in the blood and considered it holy.] These penitent parades were well planned. People volunteered for them, agreed to supply a certain amount of money per day, and the duty period was as many days as Christ lived in years.

Wherever they went, ". . . Jews were destroyed. . . ." (Brereton, 1968)[73]

As much as one third of the world's population may have died in the Great Plague.[71]

> The great plague of 1347–50 also had one positive side effect, it virtually eliminated leprosy as a major European disease. By the 1300s, leprosaria had been established throughout Europe for the isolation of infected people. When the plague struck these segregated communities of highly susceptible individuals, it completely wiped them out.[71]

I am reviewing this history in order to show how people coped with other great plagues. If you don't want this kind of coping, then do something to prevent it - and keep in mind that the law was opposed to this sort of thing. In times of social panic, the law has no effect; neither does the Church. The people take over and totally ignore conventional authority. (Serfdom was virtually obliterated by the Black Death.)

People believed that the plague was carried on the air (actually, it was carried by fleas on rats); so they would lock and guard houses for forty days - and an additional 40 days each time a new case erupted within the house. In some cases, entire families were locked up until everyone in the house died.

The confluence of American, European and African troops in World War I, and their dispersal back to their homelands in 1918–19 spread influenza worldwide. Some 20,000,000 people died of it;[70] [with this author very nearly succumbing to it in 1920–21; many in my home town did die]. "When the flu hit, medical personnel and facilities were immediately overburdened, and health services generally broke down. . . ."[70] [p. 288k]

Influenza keeps arising because it is so mutable; ". . . the brevity of the immunity it confers, and the instability of the virus that causes the disease."[70] [p. 288]

> Changes in the flu virus and mutations of other infections remains a serious possibility.[70] [p. 289]

> Even without mutation, it is always possible that some hitherto obscure parasitic organism may escape its accustomed ecological niche and expose the dense populations that have become so conspicuous a feature of the earth to some fresh and perchance devastating mortality.[70] [p. 289]

> Infectious disease which antedated the emergence of humankind will last as long as humanity itself, and will surely remain, as it has been hitherto, one of the fundamental parameters and determinants of human history.[70] [p. 291]

A PHILOSOPHER'S THOUGHTS

When humans have a problem, they use their unique ability to think, experiment, organize information and figure out what to do. But only a minute fraction of society is so engaged, while the remainder wait, suffer, die, or even go into panic. The above examples of violence were social panic. But some individuals were well disciplined - as groups, guards, executioners, etc.

In orderly society, the society has a series of recourses; which are listed and defined as follows:

1. CONSUMERS - Everybody. They use up someone else's products;

2. DISTRIBUTORS - They make someone else's products available to consumers through time and space. They deliver or distribute goods and services;

3. PRODUCERS - Final organization of all necessary aspects or components that constitute usable products or services;

4. DEVELOPERS - They take things and ideas and render them in orderly forms with methods suitable for production;

5. APPLIED RESEARCHERS - They deal in application and organization of knowledge to the point of being useful;

6. BASIC RESEARCHERS - Answer questions;

7. PHILOSOPHERS - Pose questions; and

8. "QUESTION REALIZER" - Realizes that questions of some new sort can be asked.

In World War II, the situation became so desperate that the United States realized that no existing knowledge sufficed to assure its survival. The ultimate recourse was to a Philosopher - Albert Einstein; and the answer came out to be the Atomic Bomb.

The U.S. could have won the war; but I was told that there would be a million U.S. casualties acquired in invading and conquering Japan. Indeed, Japan would have had countless more casualties in an ordinary invasion than they had from two Atomic Bombs.

So people may not like what they get by taking ultimate recourse back to Philosophers or "Question Realizers." Politicians have taken billions of dollars from hostile taxpayers and consigned them to "get the answer to the AIDS/HIV problem."

Money is not just paper - not even redeemable in anything of intrinsic value - because of acts of those who like to think of themselves as in charge. Only people do things.

We took recourse to Distributors (Hospitals, Pharmacies, Doctors, Nurses, etc.) by sending them the Consumers (AIDS patients). They could not cure AIDS/HIV. They could only ease the inevitable death.

The Distributors took recourse to Producers - but they had nothing that they could sell that would cure. Sure, they had some things for sores, pain, fever, etc. - but nothing to cure AIDS/HIV.

The Distributors have taken recourse back to Producers -but they do not know what to produce to cure AIDS/HIV.

Society has taken recourse back to Applied Research - but these people have no knowledge that applies to this new retrovirus. You can't design a vaccine with present knowledge, when this virus shows as its early symptom the destruction of the very immune system which a vaccine is intended to evoke.

We have taken recourse back to Basic Research, and a flood of knowledge pours forth. Man now knows more about this enemy than he has ever known about any enemy before. People know every molecule - every atom - that composes the virus.

But Man doesn't know how the virus works, because he doesn't understand what it acts on - Man! You see, as an example, knowing all about the nature of a bullet: Its weight, its density, its chemical composition, etc., tells you nothing about how the bullet would react with Man. The two together constitute the "system." It is necessary to understand both the HIV virus and Man, if the disease is to be understood.

Let me guess. If Man conquers AIDS/HIV, he will have gained access to knowledge which will be more disruptive to society than having one-half the population of the world die.

For example, the breakdown of the legal system of Serfdom; the religious aspects of the Black Death: A vengeful God; an "immoral" Priesthood, whipping themselves by (Church forbidden) Penitents to a bloody mess; involvement and humanitarianism and forgiveness; and other "sociological" concerns of the bubonic plague resolved themselves down to a bacterium - Pasteurella pestis, transmitted by fleas from rats. The disease is easily cured by antibiotics.[70]

Priests' prayers were not answered. It was the work of scientists that finally supplied the answer; and to that extent, Faith was badly damaged by the answer.

Nobody has the slightest clue as yet as to what institutions will cease to exist as a sequel to AIDS/HIV. Medicine? Money? Government? Religion (especially Islam - which does not even concede that Muslims can have AIDS)? African Blacks? Civilization? Some combination of the above? Time will tell.

Basic Researchers will keep grinding out knowledge according to the questions posed, and the knowledge will lead to further understanding - which is the ultimate condensation of knowledge.

But Basic Researchers don't really know the right questions, because science is composed of answers to simple questions. Even mathematics and statistics work in independent variables.

Compared with biology, all of Man's tools for understanding are too simple. The biologist, who works with the most complex things in the universe, knows those things rather than understanding them.

His grasp of biological truth is the intellectual equivalent of a taboo (i.e., knowledge) compared with the intellectual equivalent of relativity (i.e., understanding).

So the Basic Researcher must take recourse to Philosophers, who, in turn, must ask the questions that can result in the research that will give rise to the knowledge that can be used to generate the products that can be distributed to the Consumers who want to control this horrible plague.

Raising the salaries of Philosophers doesn't give rise to better thoughts.

The length of time required to go from questions like: "How many angels can dance on the head of a pin?" to: "How can there be a Science of Complexity?" could be much more than a mere 2000 years. It might, however, be sooner.

We are not upon the time when AIDS/HIV will be conquered; and it doesn't really matter what asinine politician "demands" results; nor what political activist "boos" the President because he has not complied with the whims of the uninformed.

There is work to be done, and a lot of Man's finest are dying of AIDS/HIV instead of doing the work.

Maybe the children will be shocked to see millions of their elders and contemporaries dying. One person, somewhere, may be as alienated as that German/Jew who reputedly flunked math - Albert Einstein. He had the thoughts in 1905 that led to nuclear energy in 1945 when the U.S. turned to him for the crucial questions, which resulted in the atomic bomb which ended World War II.

Maybe such an alienated child, if he can avoid being confined as insane (because of his intelligence), murdered in some extremist society, or burned at the stake - maybe he can ask the right questions to induce some humans to think in such a way that AIDS/HIV can be cured. That will probably take a while.

Meanwhile, people are trying everything they know how to do. For example, "The Search for Vaccines" is thoroughly reviewed in the special AIDS issue of *Chemical and Engineering News* (November 23, 1987) Vol. 65, No. 47. Rudy M. Baum's article reviews animal models, vaccine strategies, cytotoxic lymphocytes and subunit vaccines. Despite expert efforts: "People develop AIDS and die anyway." (Baum, 1987)[74]

Surgeon General Koop is reported to have said on CNN News on 7 January 1988 that there will never be a vaccine for AIDS. [I am blessed by having people from all over the world sending me books, journals, magazines, clippings and calling to tell me what they saw on

TV or heard on radio. I am extremely grateful, and feel humble about their help. IB]

There is always hope for a vaccine, but that must be distinguished from expectations.

DIAGNOSTICS

In a perfect world, a person infected with human immunodeficiency virus (HIV) would always show up positive in a blood test; an uninfected person would always show up negative. What could be simpler?

Unfortunately, life is not simple.

Blood banks and other HIV testing centers in the U.S. currently can choose from seven ELISA test kits that have been approved for commercial use by the Food & Drug Administration. (Dagani, 1987)[75]

Those assays test for "antibodies" - the submicroscopic units generated by Man to fight "antigens" - use the germ enemy.

"All of our data show that envelope antibody is the earliest and most important marker for detecting HIV antibody," says Rod N. Raynovich.[75] (Dagani, 1987)[75]

The massive assault on determining the presence and perhaps the quantity of HIV or its by-products will ultimately reveal accurately who had AIDS/HIV at a very early stage. If we can figure out what to do, an early test will permit us to do it.

DRUG THERAPY

Dozens of experimental drugs, including AL-721, are being tested as possible antiviral or immune-restoring agents. Some show promise. But several agents that looked promising in early tests, such as suramin, have already fallen by the wayside, or are about to. (Dagani, 1987)[76]

Azidothymidine (AZT) is the only approved therapy, and even it has toxic side effects. It retards the progression of AIDS. It costs almost $10,000 for a year's supply for one patient.[76]

According to Martin S. Hirsch (Harvard Medical School): "Never have so many antiviral drugs been developed this rapidly and never have so many clinical trials been begun for viral disease so rapidly."[76]

Critics of every stripe harass researchers: The government and all other critics operating from a basis of ignorance while not getting what they want only do harm. Research is slow and difficult, as the critics have no particular reason to know. Critics seem to think that distraction and harassment will make researchers work faster. Knowledge, unlike AIDS, is hard to get. Delay will kill more people. But maybe it doesn't matter: I think half the people in the world are going to die of it anyway.

"The NIH is not going to bow to a constituency group pushing a drug that they consider wonderful but that has been rejected by scientists," Maureen W. Myers, Chief of NIAID's (National Institute of Allergy & Infectious Diseases) Treatment Branch, said. She asserts: "Our priorities have to be based on valid scientific [considerations]."[76]

The evaluation of drugs has (according to Hirsch) three pitfalls:[76]

- "In-vitro efficacy does not necessarily predict clinical efficacy."
- "A claim of efficacy is not a demonstration of efficacy."
- "A bad clinical study is worse than no study at all."

There is one way to do good research: Slowly!

Critics and protestors who interfere are simply taking valuable time. Time kills AIDS victims. Every minute that critics waste of people who are actually doing something will probably end up killing an AIDS victim somewhere. Science is not democratic. If you're not helping, you're harmful.

According to Merle A. Sande, Chief of Medical Services at San Francisco General Hospital: "Nothing that we know of really works for this awful disease."[76]

Money has been thrown at AIDS. "The median cost of treating an AIDS victim until death is now about $75,000. (*The Economist*, 1987)[77] About 30,000 have died in the U.S. $1 billion was spent for AIDS care in the U.S. last year.[77] Not a single life was saved - illnesses were only prolonged.

I expect, as explained below, about 120,000,000 will die in the U.S. The product $1.2 \times 10^8 \times 75{,}000 = \$9{,}000{,}000{,}000{,}000$.

For whatever reason, the survivors will not spend $9 trillion.

Money, it seems, is not a problem. In the U.S., the government is allocating huge sums to AIDS research - though as the Nixon administration found in making a cure for cancer a political objective - throwing money at a disease is not necessarily a solution. (Jackson, 1987)[78]

OTHER EFFORTS TO COPE

A Texas team ". . . demonstrated that the combination of a nontoxic dye and laser light can destroy a number of viruses in blood, including the AIDS virus . . . ." (Associated Press, 1987)[79]

"Alexandria will join a growing number of cities nationwide that are responding to the AIDS crisis by requiring their firefighters and ambulance workers to wear rubber gloves on emergency calls." (Lacey, 1987)[80]

"The Indian health ministry has announced that all foreigners intending to stay for more than a year in India will have to undergo tests for AIDS. . . ." (*Nature*, August, 1987)[81]

Promise to be celibate for a year?

"U.S. Congress debates legislation in response to AIDS." (Palca, 1987)[82]

"Health Workers Given AIDS Guidelines." (Associated Press, 1987)[83]

"To prevent the transmission in health-care settings of the virus causing AIDS . . ." ". . . CDC recommended that blood and other body fluids 'from all patients' be treated as potentially infective." (Palca, 1987)[84]

The increased demand for latex gloves has caused serious shortages in dental supply stores . . . ." (Tofani, 1987)[85]

"Proposed South Africa Law Would Force Isolation of AIDS Victims." (Parks, 1987)[86]

"Meat, Poultry Inspectors With Disease Would Be Dismissed." (Sugerman, 1987)[87]

". . . virtual quarantine for Cubans known to be infected." ". . . widespread testing of the Island's [Cuba] 10 million population." (Thompson, 1987)[88]

". . . Education Secretary William J. Bennett . . . issued a guide to AIDS education that frowns on condoms and emphasizes the teaching of morality. . . ." (Associated Press, 1987)[89]

"There is considerable controversy over balancing the patient's and the health-care worker's rights." (Scott, 1988)[90]

"The British Health Department said this week that doctors with AIDS should be allowed to continue practicing except in special circumstances and that patients do not have the right to be told. . . ." (Lohr, 1987)[91]

"U.S. Will Require Health Industry to Protect Workers Against AIDS." (Pear, 1987)[92]

"AIDS-Infected Teacher Back In Classroom." . . . 9th U.S. Circuit Court of Appeals . . . American Civil Liberties Union Attorneys. . . . (Associated Press, 1987)[93]

"An empty white building beside a busy freeway is all that remains of the nation's first private hospital for AIDS patients. . . ." Houston (Associated Press, 1987)[94]

"Police Get Guidelines on AIDS" from the Justice Department - Washington. (*The New York Times*, 1987)[95]

". . . Bavaria last month put into effect some of the stiffest AIDS regulations yet ordered anywhere in the world." (Schmemann, 1987)[96]

"There have been only a handful of AIDS cases reported in China and just three confirmed deaths." (Southerland, 1987)[97]

"Indeed there is a growing concern among many health officials that the protection afforded by condoms has been exaggerated." (Seligmann and Gosnell, 1987)[98]

Governments have been counting deaths as in any plague. Thus, the U.S. government reports:

AIDS CASES

Reported - 4 January 1988

YEAR	NEW CASES	DOUBLING TIME - MONTHS
1985	8,300	
1986	13,008	21.18
1987	20,620	20.53

The 1987 figure seems speeded up because the broadening of conditions of definitions of AIDS added to the total number.

MORE EVIDENCE

A paper issued by Catholic Bishops ". . . gave qualified endorsement to teaching in Catholic institutions that condoms prevent AIDS." (Goldman, 1987)[100]

A wave of purposeful dissemination of AIDS virus by its victims had produced near panic in Brazil, but so far has not sparked violence. (Graham, 1987)[101]

"California health officials will distribute $7,600,000 . . ." to help pay the cost of AZT for AIDS victims. (*Los Angeles Times*, 1987)[102]

". . . 17 states and the District of Columbia now . . ." requires AIDS education. (Connell, 1987)[103]

"Rocky Mountain residents ranked below the national average in their own support for virtually all types of government spending but particularly for research into acquired immune deficiency syndrome and assistance to the unemployed." (Associated Press, 1987)[104]

Three hemophiliac children in Arcadia, Fla. with AIDS were ordered reinstated in school. The school was boycotted, then their house burned. The family fled, and the entire family situation was publicized by Congress. (*Chicago Tribune* Wires, 1987)[105]

The health services minimize the danger of transmission of AIDS by mosquitoes. They even deny it - which is false science. (Kotulak, 1987)[106] There is no scientific way to prove that something cannot happen.

The correct statement was made by Dr. Howard Striecher, a member of the National Cancer Institute team that is participating in the research:

> There's nothing to support the role of mosquitoes transmitting the virus to people. . . . These findings don't eliminate the theoretical possibility that a mosquito could infect someone, but it's not likely to happen.[106]

That is: The probability is low per bite.

> Such transmission may depend on the arthropod's being interrupted while feeding on one host and completing its meal on another (an event whose likelihood increases if the insect's bite is painful), on the frequency with which the arthropod takes a meal, on the size of its mouthparts, on the level of virus circulating in the host's blood, on the physical distance between successive hosts, and even on the lon-

gevity or relative abundance or distinctive feeding habits of the arthropod . . .[30]

Of course the probability is low. The number of people carrying the AIDS virus is only one to two million in the U.S. But it is going up, up, up. So there's a bigger chance (probability) of a mosquito biting you after biting an AIDS/HIV carrier.

It has been estimated that sexual intercourse with an AIDS/HIV carrier has a 1% risk of infection.

But mosquito bites are more frequent in some places than sexual intercourse.

So what probability of AIDS/HIV infection from a mosquito bite? 0.01%? 0.001%?

Let's guess 0.001%. A thousand bites, and you have one per cent, if AIDS/HIV is rampant in your neighborhood. And you get a thousand bites or so per year in mosquito country.

What is my message? Avoid insect bites - but then, who doesn't? The risk is not zero. It is real and increasing.

It is "extremely improbable" that AIDS can be spread from person to person by mosquitoes . . ." (Associated Press, 1987)[107] Right! But it is increasing and the probability per bite must be multiplied by the number of bites; and there is a wild mutation rate of the AIDS/HIV virus with unpredictable consequences.[42]

But now, enough references. Surely 107 references (plus more than a hundred more that were read but not cited) assures the reader that this author has done his homework. So what are the conclusions?

CONCLUSIONS

The genetics of people set up not only body fluids' immune system, but also a set of barriers which counter the attacks of the outside world. As these barriers are evaded, or penetrated, and the immune system itself is challenged, the probability of infection rises.

Normal monogamous sex carries a 50% probability of transmission from an AIDS/HIV carrier to his or her spouse (sole sexual partner). If neither carries the virus, then there is no sexual risk of acquiring the virus.

If sex is not strictly vaginal, the risk is higher, if one tests (+).

Anal or oral sex addresses tissues which are not genetic barriers, hence the risk increases.

Multiple partner sex (including prostitution) is high risk sex.

Use of condoms reduces but does not eliminate risk of transmission of AIDS/HIV. The risk of AIDS/HIV transmission when using condoms is about double the risk of pregnancies. Many people with families have used condoms as contraceptives - but they also have families.

Some races and ethnic groups have a much higher rate of AIDS/HIV than others.

The formula for avoiding AIDS/HIV sexually is this:

1. Marry [actual or common law] as virgins, or after having a moratorium on sex for three years;

2. Test to certainty for the presence of AIDS/HIV (in association with the three-year moratorium - to take care of the latency period);

3. Be monogamous.

Since I realize that many will not choose to do these things and do not now have an AIDS/HIV-free monogamous relationship, please let me take this opportunity to wave goodbye!

Intravenous drug abusers (dirty needles) are mostly going to die. That's "barrier breaking."

The period of latency makes blood transfusions suspect until the virus (not the antibody) has been tested.

Practice diligent hygiene.

Low probability transmission: Kissing, having someone sneeze at you, getting in crowds, bug bites, human contact, etc., are all just that; low probability. Every instance is another low probability. Enough low probabilities is a high probability.

Go, now, with my best wishes, and live carefully and long, too!

APPENDICES

APPENDIX A

CORPORATE SECURITY & INVESTIGATIONS, INC.
DESIGNING A CORPORATE AIDS POLICY

This year, according to the World Health Organization, the number of AIDS cases will double. Already, according to estimates of the Center for Disease Control, as many as 1.5 million people in the United States are infected.

In an Allstate/*Fortune* magazine survey conducted in January 1988, companies rated AIDS the third most important U.S. problem. Recent federal court rulings, based on the federal Vocational Rehabilitation Act of 1973 and various state laws, forbid employers from refusing to hire or dismissing someone because of AIDS, a defined handicap. Yet half the executives surveyed admitted their company would have an image problem if the public found out they had an employee with AIDS. Equally troublesome, over two-thirds of the workers in a nationwide survey conducted by the Center for Work Performance Problems at Georgia Institute of Technology would be afraid of acquiring AIDS from sharing restrooms with an AIDS infected co-worker. Forty per cent were concerned about using the same cafeteria and thirty seven per cent would not be willing to use the same equipment.

Besides the specter of labor unrest and a tarnished corporate image, the modern executive has to examine the bottom line impact of AIDS on his company's already growing health care costs. The insurance industry had to pay $200 million in benefits for AIDS care in 1987, which amounted to about one per cent of its total benefit outlay. Because of these increases in benefits, the 1988 premiums for major health insurance carriers will increase by 15 to 40 per cent. Although the increases in medical insurance premiums cannot totally be blamed on AIDS, it is fast becoming a significant factor of health care costs. What will costs expand to by 1991 when medical costs for AIDS are expected to go up eight-fold to $8.5 billion dollars, as predicted by William D. Grant, chairman of Business Men's Assurance Company of America?

The modern executive has two options. He can attempt to avoid the issue and wait until his company actually experiences an AIDS case with it's resulting labor unrest, lawsuits, and soaring insurance premiums, or he can use intelligent risk management techniques and create an AIDS management policy before the crisis erupts.

Corporate Security & Investigations suggests that your company consider the following issues when designing a company AIDS policy.

APPENDIX A

LEGAL ISSUES

The most important single law affecting the AIDS issue is the Vocational Rehabilitation Act of 1973 which forbids employee discrimination on the basis of physical disability by federal agencies, contractors or subcontractors receiving up to $2,500 in federal aid. (29 U.S.C. 763-764). An employer can lawfully dismiss an employee if the handicap:

1. Substantially interferes with the person's ability to perform the job after the employer has made a reasonable accommodation;

2. would pose a reasonable probability of substantial harm to others.

In the U.S. Supreme Court Case of School Board of Nassau County vs. Arline 107 S. Ct. 1123 (1987), infectious diseases were interpreted as a protected handicap. A subsequent ruling, Chalk vs. Orange County Department of Education, by the Ninth Circuit Court of Appeals extended this definition to AIDS. As such, an employer is forbidden to discriminate against an applicant or employee due to "ignorance or capitulation to public prejudice" about the person's condition.

A second relevant federal law is the Employee Retirement Income Security Act which forbids discharging or discriminating against employees for the purpose of interfering with their right to claim benefits under an employee benefit plan. This may be applicable if an employee makes an employment decision about any person with AIDS, AIDS Related Complex, or belonging to an AIDS high risk group in order to avoid incurring health care benefit claims to which an employee would be entitled under an ERISA-qualified program. (See 29 U.S.C. 1140)

Under the provisions of the federal Labor Management Relations Act, the Occupational Safety and Health Administration (OSHA), and the California state equivalent of OSHA, separate hearings have confirmed that employees who attempt to avoid contact with AIDS victims which would normally be part of their job routine can be disciplined, and even lose their jobs.

Numerous states have Handicapped Protection laws, several of them very similar in wording to the federal Vocational Rehabilitation law. It is probable that most state court systems will base their interpretations of these laws on the example set by the U.S. Supreme Court. Only Arizona, Delaware, Puerto Rico and the Virgin Islands do not have Handicapped Protection laws. Thus far, the laws in Alabama, Arkansas, Idaho, Mississippi, and South Dakota apply only to public employees.

A few cities including Austin, Texas, Los Angeles, San Francisco, Oakland, West Hollywood and Berkeley in California have local ordinances which expressly prohibit discrimination in employment against a person with AIDS, unless the employer can show that absence of AIDS is a realistic occupational qualification.

A growing number of states, Texas, California, Florida, Massachusetts and Wisconsin either ban or regulate testing job applicants for AIDS. San Francisco specifically bans testing for AIDS, while Los Angeles, San Francisco, Austin and Philadelphia have ordinances forbidding discrimination against job applicants with AIDS, ARC or carrying the HIV virus.

Finally, the District of Columbia prohibits insurers from testing for AIDS while California allows them to test only for disorders of the immune system, not for the HIV antibody. Hawaii, Rhode Island, Tennessee, Washington, New Mexico, Massachusetts and New York have similar bills pending.

PRE-SCREENING OF JOB APPLICANTS

Unless an employer can show that the absence of AIDS is a bona fide occupational qualification, it is wisest not to screen directly for AIDS. Besides being illegal in certain states and localities, it violates the federal Vocational Rehabilitation Act of 1973 if your firm is receiving federal monies. Furthermore, the most affordable tests, the ELISA and the Western Blot have both false positives and negatives. Incorrectly informing an applicant that he or she has AIDS could potentially lead to litigation.

A legal alternative is to screen for substance abuse. The latest Center for Disease Control (CDC) estimates show that intravenous drug users make up between one fifth to one fourth of the AIDS population and have the fastest spreading rate of infection. Unlike other high risk groups, however, practicing drug addicts are not protected by law.

REASONABLE ACCOMMODATION

Employers are obliged by the federal Vocational Rehabilitation Act of 1973 and most state Handicapped Protection laws to provide "reasonable accommodation" to handicapped employees on a case by case basis. This means that a company is expected to modify working conditions in order to allow a qualified employee with AIDS to perform the essential tasks of a particular job. The legal term reasonable depends on the size of the company, nature of industry and cost of the accommodation. Modifications may range from reducing the workload, to altering the work environment, to giving sick leaves necessary for treatment.

CONFIDENTIALITY

Under no circumstances may an employer reveal an employee's confidential medical record without the employee's written permission or the service of a legal subpoena. Publicly revealing an employee's condition, either through open discussions or written memos can open an employer to a defamation suit.

HARASSMENT

If an employer becomes aware of other employees isolating or harassing an employee with AIDS/HIV, they must attempt to end the activity. Otherwise the employer may legally become liable for the harassment.

PHYSICIAN VERIFICATION

Given the terms of the federal Vocational Rehabilitation Act, the employer has the right to require a physician's statement that the continued presence at work will pose no threat to the employee, co-workers or customers.

POLICY IMPLEMENTATION

One person or department should be assigned responsibility for coordinating and implementation of the adopted policy. The supervisors and employees should be advised where to direct their questions and concerns.

APPENDIX A

CO-WORKER EDUCATION

Surgeon General C. Everett Koop recommends that employers "have a plan in operation for the education of the work force before the first case of AIDS appears." A company's methods of education may vary from letters, posters, and brochures, to full scale workshops. The education process should be mandatory for all employees and include referrals to reliable sources of information. Employees need to be informed of the best medical opinions regarding the manner in which the disease can and cannot be transmitted.

If workers use needles or other instruments that penetrate the skin, or if they are health care workers in a company clinic, they should be instructed to follow the special guidelines for health care workers as established by the Center for Disease Control (CDC).

The compassionate corporate manager will not allow employees who fear getting AIDS from a co-worker to be transferred, instead they should be counseled. Indeed, arbitration hearings in Minnesota and California have taken the position that co-workers' legal rights in these situations are very limited and their continued protestations over working with an AIDS infected employee could lead to disciplinary action.

HOUSECLEANING

The Georgia Institute of Technology study revealed that restrooms, the cafeteria and shared equipment (especially masks and breathing apparatus) are areas of special concern for employees; corporate policy should emphasize cleanliness in these areas. As an additional concession to a concerned workforce, cleansing procedures might include using household bleach, which kills the AIDS virus, according to the CDC, and sterilization procedures where possible. Housekeeping staff should use gloves when cleaning up any body fluids, whether from an AIDS victim or any other worker.

INSURANCE
Creating An AIDS Policy

The formulation of a corporate policy should address a number of issues that we have already discussed:

APPENDIX A

1. A company is safer from accusations of AIDS discrimination if they create a policy for catastrophic, or long term debilitating illness and include guidelines for AIDS within that policy. Whenever possible, AIDS should be treated as any other long term illness.

2. The policy should specifically state that the corporation intends to comply with all city, state, and federal statutes that forbid discrimination. To that end, the employees must be advised of what could constitute discrimination on their part. The policy should further state that any form of discrimination directed towards any other employee for any reason will not be tolerated and may subject the violating employee to disciplinary action.

3. The medical facts relative to the manner the AIDS virus is transmitted should be specifically stated. Emphasis should be placed on known medical facts. It should be stressed that medical authorities do not believe the virus can be transmitted by casual contact.

4. Emphasis should be made that the AIDS infected person, or any worker suffering with terminal illness, should be treated fairly and with all possible consideration.

5. In corporations which involve union employees, the union should be urged to give direction to its members to fairly treat AIDS infected workers. Management should hold discussions with union representatives to urge this cooperative action.

6. A corporation should do all in its power to assist the AIDS infected employee as it would in any life-threatening illness. However, the company has the right to require minimum standards of performance and attendance be met. The company also needs to consider the safety of co-workers and customers and may find it necessary at times to require the attending physician to produce an affirmative statement. The letter must state that the continued presence of an AIDS affected employee at work will not endanger co-workers or customers. The company also may require the affected employee be examined by a company designated physician for confirmation.

7. The size of the company, the type of service rendered, the size of the work force, and the specific job requirements may all be considered in dealing with the AIDS infected employee. A company must not discriminate because a person is infected, but does have the right to protect its company and employees from

APPENDIX A

debilitating financial loss if the affected employee cannot meet acceptable standards.

The affected employee should be counseled in these circumstances and appraised as to any benefits available to disabled employees pursuant to the company policies and existing coverage.

Our legal and medical experts have approved the materials as you see them, but we caution you to check with your own authorities before you use or implement any of the materials. They will need to be modified to fit your local conditions. WE CANNOT BE RESPONSIBLE FOR ANY CLAIMS ARISING FROM YOUR USE OF THESE MATERIALS.

We thank Evelyn Garriss, Research Director for Corporate Security and Investigations, Inc., for permission to print *Designing a Corporate AIDS Policy.*

APPENDIX B

CHEVRON
JANUARY 1986
GUIDELINES FOR HANDLING
ISSUES RELATED TO AIDS

Chevron recognizes that Acquired Immune Deficiency Syndrome (AIDS) is a life-threatening illness. Due to the nature of the disease, concern continues to build worldwide.

It is further recognized that employees with AIDS, as with other life-threatening illnesses, may wish to continue to engage in as many of their normal activities, including work, as their condition permits. As long as employees with AIDS are able to meet acceptable performance and attendance standards and medical evidence indicates that their condition and actions pose no threat to the health and safety of themselves or others, efforts should be made to treat them as other employees with defined illnesses. Chevron also recognizes that it has the responsibility of providing a safe work environment for all of its employees. In view of this, every effort should be made to ensure that any employee illness, including AIDS, does not pose a health or safety risk to other employees. Consistent with the above, the following guidelines should be used throughout the company for dealing with AIDS-related employment issues:

1. Recognize that medical information is personal and confidential and take all reasonable steps to assure strict confidentiality.

2. Be sensitive to employees' concerns about AIDS and make educational material on this condition readily available to them. Contact Medical Services or Human Resources for available educational materials if you believe you or your employees need information on AIDS.

3. Contact Medical Services if you become aware that an employee has or may have AIDS. Medical Services will obtain the necessary medical information to determine if the employee is able to continue working without threat to the health and safety of the employee or co-workers.

4. Remember, when dealing with employees who have AIDS, that they may be covered by the laws and regulations that protect handicapped people against discrimination. Additionally, some cities have passed laws specifically prohibiting discrimination

against employees with AIDS. The Human Resources staff should be consulted before making any employment decisions regarding an employee with AIDS.

5. Be sensitive to the fact that employment for an individual with AIDS can be an important factor in determining the quality of life for that individual.

6. Advise employees who are known to have AIDS that information on and referral to agencies and organizations which offer supportive services for this condition are available through the Medical Services' Employee Assistance Program.

7. Advise employees who are known to have AIDS that consultation on disability plans and other benefits to assist them is available through Human Resources.

We thank CHEVRON for permission to print their policy.

APPENDIX C

THE BANK OF AMERICA
OCTOBER 1985
POLICY ON ASSISTING EMPLOYEES WITH
LIFE-THREATENING ILLNESSES

BankAmerica recognizes that employees with life-threatening illnesses including but not limited to cancer, heart disease, and AIDS may wish to continue to engage in as many of their normal pursuits as their condition allows, including work. As long as these employees are able to meet acceptable performance standards, and medical evidence indicates that their conditions are not a threat to themselves or others, managers should be sensitive to the conditions and ensure that they are treated consistently with other employees. At the same time, BankAmerica has on obligation to provide a safe work environment for all employees and customers. Every precaution should be taken to insure that an employee's condition does not present a health and/or safety threat to other employees or customers.

Consistent with this concern for employees with life-threatening illnesses, BankAmerica offers the following range of resources available through Personnel Relations:

- Management and employee education and information on terminal illnesses and specific life-threatening illnesses.

- Referral to agencies and organizations which offer supportive services for life-threatening illnesses.

- Benefit consultation to assist employees in effectively managing health, leave, and other benefits.

Guidelines - When dealing with situations involving employees with life-threatening illnesses, managers should:

1. Remember that an employee's health condition is personal and confidential, and reasonable precautions should be taken to protect information regarding an employee's health condition.

2. Contact Personnel Relations if you believe that you or other employees need information about terminal illness, or a specific life-threatening illness, or if you need further guidance in managing a situation that involves an employee with a life-threatening illness.

3. Contact Personnel Relations if you have any concern about the possible contagious nature of an employee's illness.

4. Contact Personnel Relations to determine if a statement should be obtained from the employee's attending physician that continued presence at work will pose no threat to the employee, co-workers or customers. BankAmerica reserves the right to require an examination by a medical doctor appointed by the company.

5. If warranted, make reasonable accommodation for employees with life-threatening illnesses consistent with the business needs of the division/unit.

6. Make a reasonable attempt to transfer employees with life-threatening illnesses who request a transfer and are experiencing undue emotional stress.

7. Be sensitive and responsive to co-workers' concerns, and emphasize employee education available through Personnel Relations.

8. No special consideration should be given beyond normal transfer requests for employees who feel threatened by a co-worker's life-threatening illness.

9. Be sensitive to the fact that continued employment for an employee with life-threatening illness may sometimes be therapeutically important in the remission or recovery process, or may help to prolong that employee's life.

10. Employees should be encouraged to seek assistance from established community support groups for medical treatment and counseling services. Information on these can be requested through Personnel Relations or Corporate Health.

We thank Bank of America for their permission to quote their policy.

DISCLAIMER

During the past year of our writing, we have had to change our numbers and data bases several times. For example, the amount of time necessary for AIDS antibodies to show up in blood tests was changed four times in our writing during the past year:

APPENDIX C

1. AIDS "may occur as early as one week after infection and usually precedes seroconversion, which commonly occurs between 6 and 12 weeks after infection but may take as long as 8 months." (Pilot and Colebunders, 1987)

2. "[The] antibodies detected by commonly used tests may not appear for as long as a year or more in 10 to 20 per cent of gay men who were infected through sexual contact." (Kolata, 1987)

3. ". . . the recent discovery that current antibody tests may not show signs of HIV exposure for up to 23 months." (*National Underwriter*, 1987)

4. "Fifteen per cent of another group of these subjects ['Finnish men whose homosexual partners were positive for the virus'], with persistently negative standard AIDS tests, were found to have been carrying the virus for from 10 to 34 months." (Robinson, 1987)

Therefore, although this book is replete with predictions, we disclaim any responsibility or liability to any person for any loss or damage caused by errors, omissions, or our predictions whether or not such errors, omissions, or predictions result from negligence, accident, or any other cause.

A further example: The day before this book went to Donnelley's to be printed, Goodman ran an article that said, "So far, it is believed that only a dozen health workers - including a technician here at San Francisco General - have been infected on the job." (Goodman, 1988)[1] San Francisco General was the "AIDS free" hospital referred to by Dr. Walters of the Canadian Public Health Association earlier in our book. (Walters, 1987)[74]

> "The future is obscure, even to men of strong vision, and one would perhaps be wiser not to shoot arrows into it. For the arrows will surely hit targets that were never intended." (Stigler, 1984)[2]

---

[1] Ellen Goodman, "Doctors, Nurses Deserve to Know Which Patients Have AIDS," *Albuquerque Journal*, February 26, 1988, p. A4.

[2] George J. Stigler, *The Intellectual and the Marketplace*, Cambridge, Mass.: Harvard University Press, 1984, p. 43.

REFERENCES

REFERENCES FOR PART I

1. Rebello, Kathy, "Lucrative biotech war needs winner." *USA Today*, p. 1B.
2. Krieger, Lisa M., "AIDS vaccine." *San Francisco Examiner*, December 31, 1987, p. B-13.
3. Walters, Dr. David, M.A., M.D., "WORKPLACE AIDS: 'The Non-Epidemic.' " *The New Facts of Life*; An AIDS Newsletter Prepared by the Canadian Public Health Association. December 1987, Volume 1, Issue 4.
4. Associated Press, The "AIDS Fear on Rise At Work, Study Says." *Albuquerque Journal*, February 8, 1988, p. B2.
5. *The New Facts of Life*, "Nutrition and AIDS." AIDS Education and Awareness Program of the Canadian Public." December 1987, Vol. 1, Issue 4, p. 3.
6. Connell, Christopher, "Group Reports More States Mandate AIDS Education." Associated Press, *Albuquerque Journal*, December 5, 1987, p. B8.
7. Ricklefs, Roger, "AIDS Videos for Schools." *The Wall Street Journal*, November 18, 1987, p. 22.
8. Washington (UPI), "Low-Income AIDS Victims Get U.S. Help." *Los Angeles Times*, July 25, 1987, p. 35.
9. Journal Wires, "Koop Puts $16 Billion Tag on AIDS Fight." *Albuquerque Journal*, November 7, 1987, p. A3.
10. Findlay, Steve, "A 'Manhattan Project' to Vanquish the AIDS Virus?" *U.S. News & World Report*, September 21, 1987, p. 30.
11. Associated Press, "House Panel Hears Conflicting Views on AIDS Civil Rights." *Albuquerque Journal*, September 30, 1987, p. B10.
12. Anderson, Jack, and Van Atta, Dale, "CIA Mapping Progression of AIDS." *Albuquerque Journal*, December 21, 1987, p. B2.
13. Gallo, Robert C., "The AIDS Virus." *Scientific American*, January 1987, Vol. 256, No. 1, p. 56.
14. Klingholz, Reiner, "The March of AIDS." Excerpted from "Die Zeit," *World Press Review*, February 1987, p. 57.
15. Newmark, Peter, "AIDS in an African Context." *Nature*, Vol. 324 18/25, December 1986, p. 611.
16. Newmark, Peter, "AIDS in an African Context." *Nature*, Vol. 324 18/25, December 1986, p. 611; T.C. Quinn et al., *Science* 234, pp. 955–963, 1986.
17. Barnes, Deborah M., "AIDS: Statistics But FewAnswers." *Science*, Vol. 236, June 12, 1987, p. 1423.
18. Simon, Julian L., "Life on Earth is Getting Better, Not Worse." *Global Issues* 85/86, Robert Jackson, Ed. Guilford, Connecticut: The Dushkin Publishing Group, Inc., 1985, p. 13.

REFERENCES

19. Klein, Burton H., *Prices, Wages, and Business Cycles a Dynamic Theory*. New York: Pergamon Press, 1984, p. 169.
20. *Stone Company Newsletter*, The, "Happy Home." February 1988, p. 1.
21. Beck, Joan, "Work and Family: For Women, Still A Poor Fit." *Albuquerque Journal*, August 30, 1987, p. B3.
22. *Parade Magazine*, June 28, 1987, p. 16.
23. Noble, Joseph Veach, "Museum Meltdown." *ARTnews*, February 1988, p. 176.
24. Shilts, Randy, "AIDS in 1991 - A Grim Challenge for S. F." *San Francisco Chronicle*, August 3, 1987, p. 8.
25. *New York Times*, The, "Head Start on Head Start," January 13, 1987, p. Y21.
26. Associated Press, "Americans Living Better Today, Fortune Says." *Albuquerque Journal*, August 30, 1987, p. D7.
27. Clark, Kenneth R., "Captain Prospers in Mr. Rogers' Environs." *Chicago Tribune* quoted in *Albuquerque Journal*, October 30, 1987, p. H39.
28. Rostvold, Gerhard, "Economic Update: After the Downdraft." Presentation to The Executive Committee, a Chief Executive Officer's Organization, January 28, 1988.
29. Landis, David, and Guy, Pat, "Home Prices: Two Incomes To Keep Up; Our Dream Home is Shrinking." *USA Today*, February 4, 1988, pp. 1A & 4B.
30. Cox, Meg, "Crash Victims: Many Who Lost Jobs After Black Monday Still Pound Pavements." *The Wall Street Journal*, February 9, 1988, p. 1.
31. Minsky, Hyman P., "The Potential for Financial Crises." Working Paper Series, Department of Economics, Washington University, 1982, p. 17.
32. Minsky, Hyman P., *Can It Happen Again*. Armonk, New York: M. E. Sharpe & Co., 1982; and Kalecki, M., *Essays in the Theory of Economics Fluctuations*. London: Allen and Unwin, 1939.
33. Meyer, Anthony, "A New World With AIDS - Health Promotion as a Catalyst for Change." *The Western Journal of Medicine*, Vol. 114, #6.
34. *Wall Street Journal*, The, December 29, 1987, p. 1.
35. Lent, Charles M., "AIDS: Another Threat." *Nature*, Vol. 328, August 6, 1987, p. 470; and [1]III International Conference on AIDS, Washington, D. C., 1–5 June 1987.

REFERENCES

36. Chase, Marilyn, "Lab Worker Is Infected With AIDS Virus; Vigilance in Safety Measures Urged." *The Wall Street Journal*, January 4, 1988, p. 4.
37. Greene, Ralph, "Personal Autonomy and Public Health: An Ethical Imperative for Preventing Disease." *The Humanist*, July/August 1987, p. 6.
38. *Wall Street Journal, The*, "AIDS Fears Alter Medical Products." October 1, 1987, p. 1.
39. Miller, A. E., Jr., M.D., "Medical 'Miracles' Cost More Than Money." *Reader's Digest*, Condensed from AP NEWS FEATURES, December 1987, pp. 103–104.
40. Reuters, "Some Hospitals Carrying Brunt of AIDS Care." *Albuquerque Journal*, September 13, 1987, p. A14.
41. Myatt, Art, "Health Care Economics and AIDS: What's the Prognosis for our Health and Insurance Industries in a Future with AIDS?" *The Humanist*, July/August 1987, pp. 19 & 20.
42. Associated Press, *Albuquerque Journal*, February 5, 1988, p. B8.
43. Sullivan, Ronald, "AIDS Cost for New York in '91 Put At $2 Billion by State Study." 'New York News', *The New York Times*, July 9, 1987, p. Y15.
44. Schmitt, Eric, "Suburbs Straining to Build Services for AIDS Patients." *The New York Times*, August 3, 1987, p. 8.
45. Schwartz, William A., "Drug Addicts With Dirty Needles." *The Nation*, June 20, 1987, p. 843.
46. Lockwood, Charles, and Leinberger, Christopher B., "Los Angeles Comes of Age." *The Atlantic*, January 1988, pp. 35, 41, and 48.
47. Lemann, Nicholas, "Growing Pains." *The Atlantic*, January 1988, p. 58.
48. Kaplan, Helen S., *The Real Truth About Women and AIDS*. New York: Simon & Schuster, 1987.
49. Wartzman, Rick, "AIDS Heaps Hardship on Washington Slum Called 'the Graveyard.'" *The Wall Street Journal*, November 4, 1987, p. 1.
50. Engel, Mary, "Health Care for Homeless Puts Stress on the Caring." *Albuquerque Journal*, November 22, 1987, p. B3.
51. Quinn, Jane Bryant, "When It Comes To Health Insurance, AIDS Could Have Some Precedent-Setting Effects." *Chicago Tribune*, Business 2, Section 4, July 6, 1987.

REFERENCES

52. Dunea, George, "AIDS Update." *British Medical Journal*, Vol. 295, August 22, 1987, p. 492.
53. Griffin, Jean Latz, and Galvan, Manuel, "Minority Percentage of AIDS Cases Rising." *The New York Times*, August 8, 1987, p. 14.
54. Schmidt, William E., "High AIDS Rate Spurring Efforts For Minorities." *The New York Times*, August 8, 1987, p. 14.
55. Curry, George E., "More AIDS Help Urged for Blacks." *Chicago Tribune*, July 22, 1987, p. 7.
56. Boodman, Sandra G., "Hispanics' Rate of Contracting AIDS Increases." *Albuquerque Journal*, December 29, 1987, p. B3.
57. Reuters, "Test of Recruits Details Heterosexual AIDS Trend." *The Washington Post*, July 16, 1987, p. A5.
58. Taggart, Robert, *Hardship: The Welfare Consequences of Labor Market Problems*. Kalamazoo, Michigan: W. E. UpJohn Institute For Employment, 1982.
59. Murray, Dorothy F., Project Director, and Barker, Valerie C., Editor, *The Retirements Markets: Overview and Outlook*. Hartford, Conn.: Life Insurance Marketing and Research Association, Inc., 1986.
60. Fischer, Donald E., "Consumer Credit." *Encyclopedia Americana*, New York: Encyclopedia Americana Corp., 1969, Vol. 7, p. 682.
61. *The Economist*, "American Survey, The Awful Cost of AIDS." April 11, 1987, p. 21.
62. Davidson, Joe, "Medicaid Spending on AIDS to Increase Sixfold by 1992, Health Official Says." *The Wall Street Journal*, September 10, 1987, p. 12.
63. *Albuquerque Tribune, The*, "Medicare to Cover More." October 28, 1987, p. A4.
64. *AARP News Bulletin*, "How a Modest Idea Evolved Into a Watershed Bill." Vol. 29, No. 2, February 1988, p. 1.
65. Bean, Ed, "In Poor Health, Small Rural Hospitals Struggle for Survival Under Medicare Setup." *The Wall Street Journal*, January 4, 1988, pp. 1 and 6.
66. Goodman, John C., "Wrong Rx for Long-Term Health Care." *The Wall Street Journal*, December 30, 1987, p. 12.
67. Perls, Fritz, "Living Gestalt." *The Handbook of Gestalt Therapy*. New York: Jason Aronson, Inc., 1976, p. 206.
68. *Wall Street Journal, The*, December 3, 1987, p. 1.

REFERENCES

69. Sabatier, Renee C., "Social, Cultural and Demographic Aspects of AIDS." *The Western Journal of Medicine*, Vol. 147, #6, December 1987, p. 713.
70. Meyer, Anthony J., "A New World With AIDS-Health Promotion as a Catalyst for Change." *The Western Journal of Medicine*, Vol. 147, #6, December 1987, p. 716.
71. *Wall Street Journal, The*, "A National AIDS Test." September 9, 1987, p. 9.
72. Associated Press, "House Panel Hears Conflicting Views on AIDS Civil Rights." *Albuquerque Journal*, September 30, 1987, p. B 10.
73. Smothers, Ronald, "Survey Finds a Clash on AIDS in Workplace." *The New York Times*, February 7, 1988, p. 6.
74. Walters, David, M.A., M.D., "Workplace AIDS: 'The Non-Epidemic.' " *The New Facts of Life* (An AIDS Newsletter prepared by the Canadian Public Health Association), Vol. 1, Issue 4, December, 1987, p. 1.
75. *Wall Street Journal, The*, John Hancock Advertisement, January 26, 1988, p. 23.
76. *National Underwriter*, "Aggressive Marketers Will Pay Price in AIDS Claims: Study." August 17, 1987, p. 6.
77. *Albuquerque Journal*, "Insurance Industry Fears AIDS Threat." September 29, 1987, p. B5.
78. Ness, Immanuel, "ACLI Study Sets 1986 AIDS Claims at $29M." *National Underwriter*, December 21, 1987, p. 1.
79. *National Underwriter*, "AIDS is Growing Problem For Group Insurers." December 21, 1987, p. 3.
80. *Albuquerque Journal*, "Most Insurance Firms Screen for AIDS." February 18, 1988, p. A3.
81. Meyer, Anthony J., "A New World With AIDS - Health Promotion as a Catalyst for Change." *The Western Journal of Medicine*, Vol. 147, #6, December 1987, p. 716; Meyer's Reference Source: [2]Hardy, A.M., Raugh, K., Echenberg, D., et.al., "The economic impact of the first 10,000 cases of Acquired Immunodeficiency Syndrome in the United States." JAMA 1986 Jan. 10; 255:209–211.
82. *Facts on File*, November 15, 1985, p. 856.
83. *Research News*, "AIDS: Statistics But Few Answers." June 12, 1987, p. 1423.
84. Robinson, J. D., "AIDS Report in *The Lancet* Punctures Complacency." *The Wall Street Journal*, October 6, 1988, p. 20.

REFERENCES

85. *Washington Post, The*, Quoted in the *Albuquerque Journal*, "Loss of Mental Function May Be First Symptom of AIDS," December 18, 1987, p. 2.
86. U.S. Government, *Dictionary of Occupational Titles*, Fourth Edition Supplement, 1986.
87. Alsop, Ronald, "Advertisers Retreat From Making Direct Pitch to the Gay Market." *The Wall Street Journal*, January 26, 1988, p. 33.
88. *Albuquerque Journal*, "Laser 'Tongs' Trap Live Cells." January 25, 1988, p. B1.
89. Berkman, Leslie, "AIDS Causes Shortage of Disposable Surgical Gloves." *Los Angeles Times* in *Albuquerque Journal*, December 13, 1987, p. C4.
90. Associated Press, "Educate Employees On AIDS, Koop Says." *Albuquerque Journal*, October 14, 1987, p. C14.
91. Spolar, Chris, "Firms Slow to Set Policies On Employees With AIDS;" "Education Of Work Force Called Key;" "Area Firms Struggle With AIDS Issue;" "Some Settle Quietly With Fired Patients;" "Some Large Local Firms Begin AIDS Education." *The Washington Post*, September 7, 1987, pp. 1, A28, A29, A30.
92. Masi, Dale S., "AIDS in the Workplace: What Can Be Done?" *PERSONNEL*, July 1987, p. 57.
93. Myers, Phyllis Schiller, and Donald W. Myers, "AIDS: Tackling a Tough Problem Through Policy; Developing a Workplace Policy on AIDS May Be a Complex Task," *Personnel Administrator*, April 1987, p. 95.
94. Magnus, Margaret, Editor, "Employee Assistance: AIDS Information Clearinghouse Launched by Personnel Journal," *Personnel Journal*, September 1987, p. 18.
95. Elliott, Robert H., and Wilson, Thomas M., "AIDS in the Workplace: Public Personnel Management and the Law," *Public Personnel Management*, Vol. 16, #3, Fall 1987, p. 209.
96. Waldo, William S., "The Work Environment: A Practical Guide for Dealing With AIDS at Work," *Personnel Journal*, August 1987, p. 135.
97. Puckett, Sam B., "When a Worker Gets AIDS; Education is the key to preventing employee panic and fear," *Psychology Today*, January 1988, p. 26.
98. Lutgen, Lorraine, "AIDS in the Workplace: Fighting Fear with Facts and Policy," *Personnel*, November 1987, p. 53.

REFERENCES

99. Magnus, Margaret, Editor, "The Workplace & AIDS: A Guide to Services and Information," *Personnel Journal*, October 1987, p. 65.
100. Verespej, Michael A., "Dealing with AIDS; Above all, the victim needs compassion - and understanding," *Industry Week*, February 1, 1987, p. 47.
101. Ember, Lois R., "The Public Health Challenge," *Chemical & Engineering NEWS*, Vol. 65, #47, November 23, 1987, p. 50.
102. Chase, Marilyn, "Corporations Urge Peers to Adopt Humane Policies for AIDS Victims," *The Wall Street Journal*, January 20, 1988, p. 1.
103. *New York Times, The*, February 7, 1988, p. 28.
104. *Personnel Management*, "Approach to AIDS Must Tackle Prejudice," August 1987, p. 8.
105. Wermiel, Stephen, "Reagan Choices Alter The Makeup and Views of the Federal Courts," *The Wall Street Journal*, February 1, 1988, p. 1.
106. Reibstein, Larry, "Case That May Force Rigid Justification For Promotions Goes Before High Court," *The Wall Street Journal*, January 19, 1988, p. 18.
107. *Personnel Management*, "Approach to AIDS Must Tackle Prejudice." August 1987, p. 8.
108. Rees, Malcome, "The Sombre View of AIDS," *Nature*, Vol. 326/26, March 1987, p. 345.

REFERENCES FOR PART II

1. Spector, William S., Ed., *Handbook of Biological Data.** Pub. by W. B. Saunders Co., Philadelphia and London, 1956.
   *NOTE: Dr. Iben Browning Was a Contributor to This Handbook.
2. Okie, Susan, Public Health Experts Raise "Doubts On Plan To Test Immigrants For AIDS." *The Washington Post*, 1987.
3. Adler, Michael W., "ABC of AIDS: Development of the Epidemic." *British Medical Journal*, 1987, Vol. 294.
4. United States Aids Program, Center for Infectious Diseases, Centers for Disease Control, "AIDS Weekly Surveillance Report." November 2, 1987.
5. Japenza, Ann, "Longevity of Some Aids Patients Offers Hope." *Los Angeles Times*, September, 1987, Part VI.
6. McWhirter, Norris, Ed., *Guinness 1983 Book of World Records*, Pub. by Bantam Books, 1983.

REFERENCES

7. *Los Angeles Times*, "Cell That Destroys AIDS Virus Discovered." July 23, 1987.
8. *New York Times*, The, "AIDS-Infected Are Found To Produce Virus-Killers." July 23, 1987.
9. AIDS Program, Atlanta Georgia, "Revision of The CDC Surveillance Case Definition for Acquired Immunodeficiency Syndrome," Morbidity and Mortality Weekly Report, August 14, 1987, Vol. 36, No. 1S.
10. Von Reyn, Fordham C., M.D. and Mann, Jonathan M., M.D., M.P.H., Geneva, "Global Epidemiology." *AIDS-A Global Perspective*, West J. Med., 1987, Dec; 147:694–701.
11. Mortimer, P. P., "ABC of AIDS; The Virus and The Tests." *British Medical Journal*, June 20, 1987, Vol. 294.
12. Gallo, Robert C., "The AIDS Virus." *Scientific American*, January 1987.
13. Piot, Peter, M.D. and Colebunders, Robert, M.D.: "Clinical Manifestations and the Natural History of HIV Infection in Adults." *AIDS-A Global Perspective*, West J Med. December 1987; 147: 709–712.
14. Kolata, Gina, "New Finding Made on AIDS Detection: Tests May Fail to Indicate the Virus for More Than a Year." *The New York Times*, Oct. 3, 1987, Vol. CXXXVII, No. 47, p. 281.
15. Ness, Immanuel, "ACLI Study Sets 1986 AIDS Claims at $290M." *National Underwriter*, Dec. 21, 1987, No. 51.
16. *Los Angeles Times*, "Eight-Year Dormancy Seen in Blood-Linked Cases." August 20, 1987, Part I.
17. Associated Press, The, "AIDS May be Top Killer in 10 Years, Expert says." *Arizona Republic*, December 6, 1987, p. 13.
18. Reuters, "Some Hospitals Carrying Brunt of AIDS Care." *Albuquerque Journal*, Sept. 13, 1987.
19. Facts on File, 1986.
20. Dunea, George, "AIDS Update." *Letter From Chicago*, August 22, 1987.
21. Griffin, Jean Latz, "AIDS Sneaks Up On Hemophiliacs." *Chicago Tribune*, August 30, 1987, pp. 1, 14.
22. Millar, Ann, "AIDS and the Lang.": *British Medical Journal*, May 23, 1987, Vol. 294.
23. Mindel, Adrian, "ABC of AIDS; Management of Early HIV Infection." *British Medical Journal*, May 9, 1987, Vol. 294.
24. Smith, Neil & Spittle, Margaret, "ABC of AIDS; Tumors." *British Medical Journal*, May 16, 1987, Vol. 294.

REFERENCES

25. Weller, Ian V.D., "ABC of AIDS; Gastrointestinal and Hepatic Manifestations." *British Medical Journal*, June 6, 1987, Vol. 294.
26. Arndt, Cheril, "Insurers Oppose Proposed Mass. AIDS Regulation." *National Underwriters*, August 31, 1987.
27. Cimons, Marlene, "Risks of Youths Contracting AIDS Virus is Seen on Rise." *Los Angeles Times*, November 6, 1987, Part I.
28. Fisher, Mary Jane, "Government Refiguring AIDS Data." *National Underwriter*, November 23, 1987.
29. Valencis, Bill, Comp., "Table of AIDS Cases and Deaths." *Personal Communications*, November 18, 1987.
30. Leishman, Katie, "AIDS and Insects." *The Atlantic Monthly*, September 1987.
31. Browning, Iben, "Ethnicity in the U.S." *The Browning Newsletter*, November 21, 1985, Vol. 9, No. 10.
32. Browning, Iben, "Newsnotes," *The Browning Newsletter*, December 21, 1985, Vol. 9, No. 11.
33. Texas Instruments Learning Center & University Of Denver Mathematics Laboratory; Calculator Decision-Making Sourcebook, Pub. by Texas Instruments, Inc., 1977, No. 77-18314.
34. Baum, Rudy M., "The Molecular Biology." *Chemical & Engineering News*, Nov. 23, 1987, Vol. 65, No. 47.
35. *Facts on File*, "U.S. Tests of French Aids Drug OK'd." October 1985.
36. *Facts on File*, "Medicine," October 1985.
37. Van, Jon, "AIDS Virus, Nerve-Cell Link Found." *Chicago Tribune*, August 28, 1987.
38. *Facts on File*, "AIDS," November 15, 1985.
39. *Facts on File*, "AIDS," July 11, 1986.
40. Associated Press, The, "AIDS Cases May Reach 100 Million Worldwide." *Albuquerque Journal*, November 14, 1987.
41. Spice, Byron, "Rapid AIDS Mutations Could Defy Detection." *Albuquerque Journal*, September 2, 1987.
42. Rensberger, Boyce, "AIDS Virus a Clever Enemy, Study Shows." *The Washington Post*, September 6, 1987.
43. Spice, Byron, "AIDS Virus Advancing; Battle Against Disease by Rapid Pace of Genetic Mutation." *Albuquerque Journal*, September 14, 1987.
44. Wilford, John Noble, "Skeletons Record the Burdens of Work." *The New York Times*, October 27, 1987.
45. Coburn, Don, "AIDS Rap Reaches Minority Youth." *Washington Post*, October 13, 1987.

REFERENCES

46. Gargan, Edward A., "China Taking Stringent Measures to Prevent Introduction of AIDS." *The New York Times*, December 22, 1987, Vol. CXXXVII, No. 47, 361.
47. Klingholz, Reiner, "Die Zeit." *New Scientist*, February 1987.
48. Crewdson, John, "How Long Has Virus Been Stalking Victims?" *Chicago Tribune*, October 25, 1987.
49. Crewdson, John, "Case Shakes Theories of AIDS Origin." *Chicago Tribune*, October 25, 1987.
50. Okware, Samuel Ikwaras, MD, MPH, DPH, MBChB, "Towards a National AIDS Control Program in Uganda." *Western Journal of Medicine*, December 1987.
51. Browning, Iben "AIDS." *The Browning Newsletter*, December 1983, Vol. 7, No. 11.
52. Browning, Iben "AIDS." *The Browning Newsletter*, March 1984, Vol. 8, No. 2.
53. Browning, Iben, *The Browning Newsletter*, November 1986, Vol. 10, No. 10.
54. Johnstone, Bill, "German Survey's Gloomy Outlook." *Nature*, November 20, 1986, Vol. 324.
55. Newmark, Peter, "AIDS in an African Context," *Nature*, December 18/25, 1986, Vol. 324.
56. Carne, C. A., "ABC of AIDS; Neurological Manifestations." *British Medical Journal*, May 30, 1987.
57. Barnes, Deborah M., "AIDS: Statistics But Few Answers." *Research News*, June 12, 1987.
58. Rist, Curtis, "Mesquite Case Spurs New AIDS Debate; Questions Surround Health Workers." *The Dallas Morning News*, September 21, 1987.
59. Lambert, Bruce, "AIDS Deaths Soar in New York." *The New York Times*, July 18, 1987.
60. Lambert, Bruce, "On AIDS, We Have More Answers Than Questions." *The New York Times*, July 12, 1987.
61. Associated Press, The, "Army Finds AIDS Virus in 1.5 of Every 1,000 Tests." *Albuquerque Journal*, July 16, 1987.
62. Reuters, "Test of Recruits Details Heterosexual AIDS." *The Washington Post*, July 16, 1987.
63. Nelson, Harry, "AIDS Risk for Women, Young Rises." *Los Angeles Times*, July 16, 1987, Part I.
64. Kraft, Scott, "Toll Threatens Hard-Earned Gains in Nations With Meager Resources." *Los Angeles Times*, August 9, 1987.

REFERENCES

65. V.R., "AIDS Test Compulsory." *Nature*, September 3, 1987, Vol. 329.
66. Griffin, Jean Latz, and Galvan, Manuel, Minority Percentage of AIDS Cases Rising." *Chicago Tribune*, September 4, 1987.
67. *Information Please Almanac Atlas and Yearbook*, Pub. by Houghton Mifflin Company, Boston, 1988, 41st Edition.
68. United States AIDS Program, "United States Cases Reported to CDC." Oct. 12, 1987.
69. Browning, Iben, *The Browning Newsletter*, February 21, 1983, Vol. 7, No. 1.
70. McNeil, William H., *Plagues and Peoples*. Pub. by Anchor Press/Doubleday, 1976.
71. Cornell, James, *The Great International Disaster Book*. Pub. by Charles Scribner's Sons/New York, 1976.
72. Tuchman, Barbara W., *A Distant Mirror; The Calamitors 14th Century*. Pub. by Ballantine Books, 1978.
73. Brereton, Geoffrey, Ed., *Froissart Chronicles*. Pub. by Penguin Books, 1968.
74. Baum, Rudy M., "The Search for Vaccines." *Chemical & Engineering News*, November 23, 1987, Vol. 65, No. 47.
75. Dagani, Ron, "The Problem of Diagnostic Tests." *Chemical & Engineering News*, November 23, 1987, Vol. 65, No. 47.
76. Dagani, Ron, "The Quest for Therapy." *Chemical & Engineering News*, November 23, 1987, Vol. 65, No. 47.
77. *Economist, The*, "The Awful Cost of AIDS." April 11, 1987.
78. Jackson, Tony, "Search for a Drug To Fight AIDS." *World Press Review*, March 1987.
79. Associated Press, The, "Laser Rides Blood of Sex Virus." *The Arizona Republic*, January 13, 1987.
80. Lacey, Marc, "Alexandria to Require Gloves to Avoid AIDS; Fire Department Policy Follows Lead by Other Municipalities." *The Washington Post*, July 16, 1987.
81. K.S.J., "AIDS Tests in India." *Nature*, August 6, 1987, Vol. 328.
82. Dickman, Steven, and Palca, Joseph, "West Berlin to Be Site of New West German AIDS Centre;" and "U.S. Congress Debates Legislation in Response to AIDS." *Nature*, August 13, 1987, Vol. 328.
83. *Los Angeles Times*, "Health Workers Given AIDS Guidelines." August 21, 1987.
84. Palca, Joseph, "New AIDS Control Recommendations." *Nature*, August 27, 1987, Vol. 328.

REFERENCES

85. Tofani, Loretta, "Dentists Taking More Precautions Against AIDS and Other Diseases." *Albuquerque Journal*, August 28, 1987.
86. Parks, Michael, "Proposed S. Africa Law Would Force Isolation of AIDS Victims." *Los Angeles Times*, September 4, 1987.
87. Sugarman, Carole, "AIDS Policy Proposed For USDA; Meat, Poultry Inspectors With The Disease Would Be Dismissed." *The Washington Post*, September 12, 1987.
88. Thompson, Larry, "Cuba Details Massive AIDS Program; Tests of 1.1 Million Said to Detect 147 Cases." *The Washington Post*, September 16, 1987.
89. Associated Press, The, "Bennett Stresses Morality in AIDS Guide." *Albuquerque Journal*, October 7, 1987.
90. Scott, Lilli, "A Fear in the Foxholes, Health Workers' Alarm About Treating AIDS Patients." *New York*, January 4, 1988.
91. Lohr, Steve, "British Policy on Doctors With AIDS." *The New York Times*, November 20, 1987.
92. Pear, Robert, "U.S. Will Require Health Industry to Protect Workers Against AIDS." *The New York Times*, July 23, 1987.
93. Associated Press, The, "AIDS-Infected Teacher Back in Classroom." *Albuquerque Journal*, November 24, 1987.
94. Associated Press, The, "First Private AIDS Facility Closes Doors." *Albuquerque Journal*, December 11, 1987.
95. Washington-"Police Get Guidelines on AIDS." *The New York Times*, August 3, 1987.
96. Schmemann, Serge, "What to Do? Bavaria Has Some Strict Ideas." *The New York Times*, July 12, 1987.
97. Southerland, Daniel, "AIDS Victim in China to Get Military Airlift; Family Pays $40,000 for Air Force Plane." *Washington Post*, July 15, 1987.
98. Seligmann, Jean & Gosnell, Mariana, "A Warning To Women on AIDS; Counting on Condoms is Flirting With Death." *Lifestyles*, August 31, 1987.
99. Atlanta-"U.S. AIDS cases Pass 50,000 Mark." *Albuquerque Journal*, January 13, 1988.
100. Goldman, Ari F., "2 Divided Camps of Bishops Form Over Catholic AIDS Policy Paper." *The New York Times*, December 17, 1987.
101. Graham, Bradley, "Some Victims' Wish to Spread AIDS Sparks Fear in Brazil." *The Washington Post*, November 4, 1987.
102. "Money Slated for AIDS Drug." *Los Angeles Times*. October 9, 1987.
103. Cornell, Christopher, "Group Reports More States Mandating AIDS Education." *Albuquerque Journal*, December 5, 1987.

104. Associated Press, The, "Study Finds More People Disaffected in Rockies." *Albuquerque Journal*, November 12, 1987.
105. "AIDS Scare Left Family No Choice." *Chicago Tribune*, September 1, 1987.
106. Kotulak, Ronald, "Studies Reassuring on Mosquitoes, AIDS." *Chicago Tribune*, July 5, 1987.
107. Associated Press, The, "Mosquito AIDS Link Minimized." *Albuquerque Journal*, September 10, 1987.

ABOUT THE AUTHORS

Iben Browning has a Ph.D. in Physiology, with Minors in Genetics and Bacteriology. He headed the Department of Biology at M.D. Anderson Hospital, a Cancer Research Center. Therefore, he is eminently qualified to speak in biological terms.

In addition, he has been a Consultant to Mitchell - Hutchins and its successor, Paine Webber, for 13 years. Dr. Browning has dealt extensively in commodities (particularly food crops) and related financial matters. His economic background further qualifies him to make statements regarding the economic consequences of AIDS.

Dr. Browning is listed in AMERICAN MEN OF SCIENCE and WHO'S WHO IN AMERICA.

Anne Aaron is uniquely qualified to write about AIDS. She began college with an eighth grade education and graduated with Distinction, Magna Cum Laude. Although she majored in History and minored in English and Political Science, her undergraduate background was so varied that she taught science her first year of teaching. Her Master's Degree is in Language Arts, and she is presently completing her Ph.D. in Family Studies.

But far more than an eclectic intellectual, Aaron is a proven business woman. She ran a development company and is a licensed general contractor. Her private investments have been very successful. From the tried and proven perspective of a business person and social scientist, Aaron writes to you about the social and business implications of AIDS.

INDIANS AND AIDS   by Dr. Maria Fagnan,

Is AIDS going to decimate the Native American population? Or, are alarmists overstating the key issues? In this informative and enlightening book on AIDS as it affects an ethnic minority, a well-known counselor and a professional writer carefully examine the problem. Dr. Maria Fagnan is the program director at the University of New Mexico Alcohol and Drug Abuse Studies Institute and is the conference coordinator of the First National Indian AIDS Training Conference.

NEWSLETTERS

World AIDS: The Newsletter

Contributors: ANNE AARON & IBEN BROWNING
(Available: August 1988)
Monthly Newsletter
$250/Year

Economic Forecasting for Business and Investors

By ANNE AARON & GERHARD ROSTVOLD
(Available: August, 1988)
Monthly Newsletter
$250/Year

AIDS INFORMATION CHARTS

AIDS and HEALTH

5 Charts:

Known AIDS Transmission

Improbable (But Possible) Transmission

Safe Sex

The Condom Threat

Doubling Rate of AIDS

(19 x 25) $25.00
(24 x 36) $35.00

AIDS and ECONOMICS

5 Charts:

Doubling Rate of AIDS

Lost Productivity

Increasing Support Demands

AIDS Impact on Families

AIDS Impact on Business: Planning & Policies

(19 x 25) $25.00
(24 x 36) $35.00

AIDS VIDEOS

ECONOMICS OF AIDS ANNE AARON'S lecture to the Medical Community
Duration: 22 Minutes
$150.00

AIDS DISCUSSION A summary discussion of the materials in **AIDS** - An Interview with Anne Aaron and Iben Browning
Made so TV stations can substitute their own interviewer
Duration: 22 Minutes
$150.00

OTHER BOOKS & LEARNING MATERIALS FROM SAPIENS PRESS

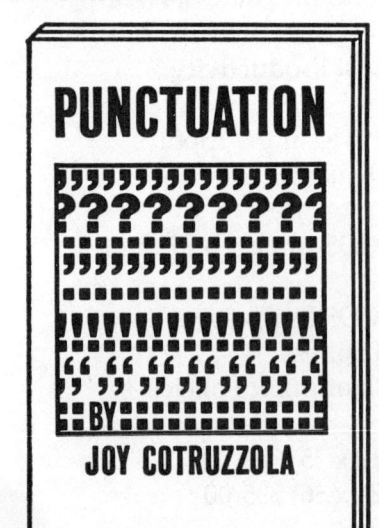

PUNCTUATION By JOY COTRUZZOLA

A complete guide to punctuation

Takes anyone 9–90 years through simple, compound, complex, and compound-complex sentences

Easy to Understand

Tested and proven in college preparatory schools and colleges

$4.95

CHALLENGES

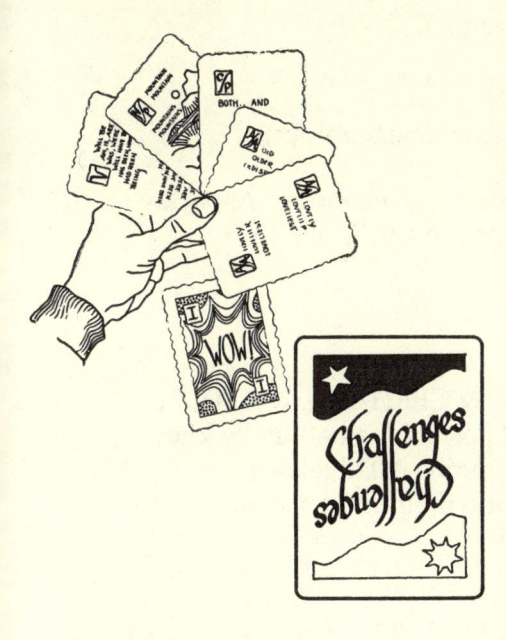

A 54-Card game that colorfully teaches grammar and syntax without any boredom

4 SUITS:
1. Noun/Pronoun
2. Verb
3. Adjective/Adverb
4. Conjunction/Preposition
   2 Exclamations!

Tested and proven
Grade school children and professors have played this game and loved it

FUN!

Two Different Decks,
54 Cards Each &
Guide Rules

$12.95

COMING SOON

AIDS: ACTIONS for AMERICANS

> By ANNE AARON
> (Available Summer)
>
> Health, Social, and Economic Aspects of AIDS (not a rerun; ALL NEW)

AIDS and BUSINESS

> By ANNE AARON & GERHARD ROSTVOLD
> Aaron and Rostvold, a nationally known economist, probe AIDS related problems and their influence on BUSINESS

---------------------------------- (DETACH HERE) ----------------------------------

Sapiens Press • 2430 Juan Tabo N.E. • Suite 256 • Albuquerque, NM 87112

Name: _____

Address: _____

City: _____

State: _____ Zip: _____

Check or Money Order
(Charge Orders $15 Minimum)

VISA # _____

MASTERCARD # _____
Card Expiration Date: _____

Please add $3.00 for shipping & insurance for book orders. For book orders of 100 or more copies, please call for discount schedule — (505) 888-3766. Allow 6 weeks for delivery.